Basic Client Care

Charlene Thiessen | Russell Jordan II

Second Edition

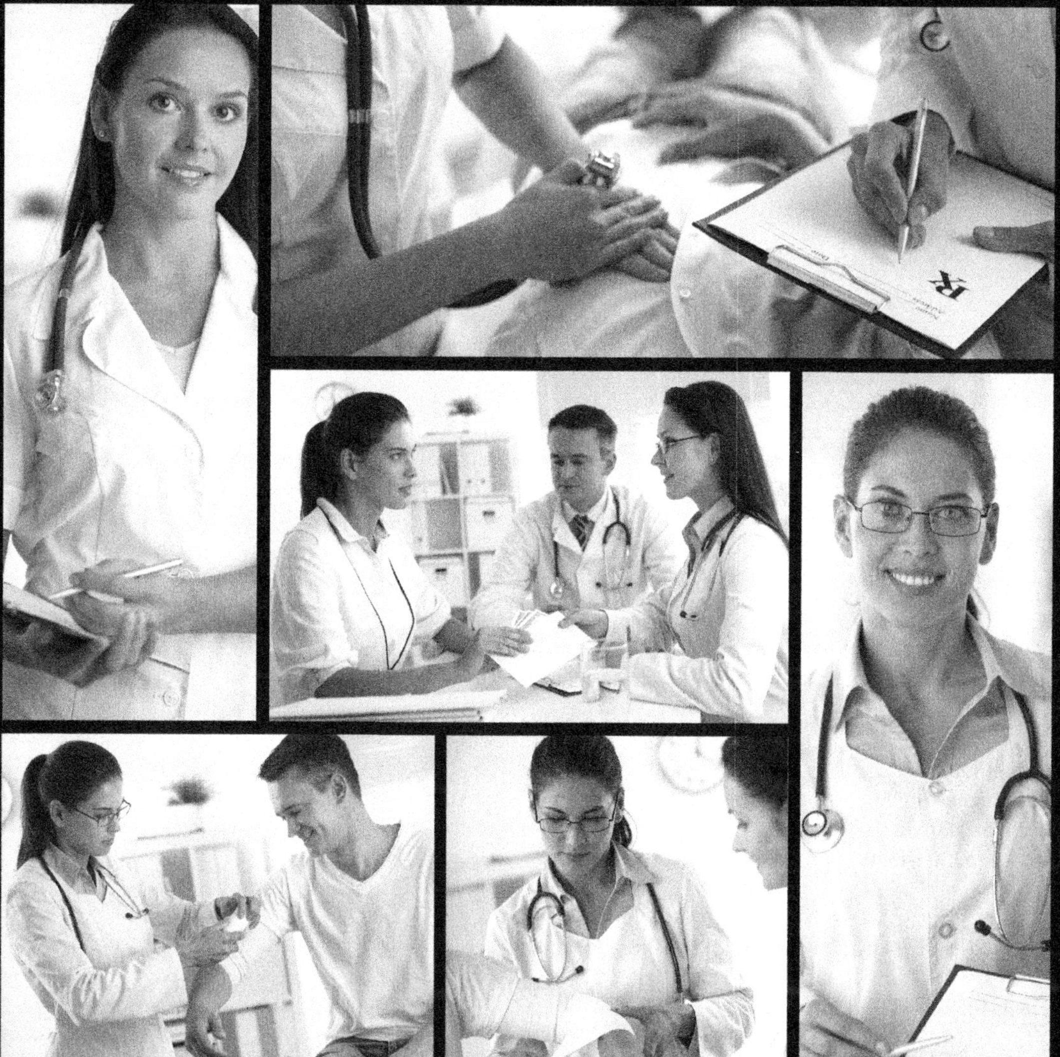

Kendall Hunt
publishing company

Cover images: Used under license of Shutterstock, Inc.

Kendall Hunt
publishing company

www.kendallhunt.com
Send all inquiries to:
4050 Westmark Drive
Dubuque, IA 52004-1840

Contents

Preface

The collaborative work of the Basic Client Care 2nd Edition has been reworked to enhance student and individual's knowledge that have an interest and appreciation in starting a healthcare career. The contents have been expanded to encompass an in-depth understanding of the essentials of care and a platform from which to develop an educational allied health understanding. This book has been developed to meet the course requirements for Maricopa Community Colleges. Additional exercises and activities have been provided to increase reader understanding and application awareness.

Acknowledgments

Charlene Thiessen

Thanks to my husband for his encouragement and support in the process of writing this book. Thanks to Gwen Bilek for providing me with the inspiration for this book. Her input helped me get started with the writing.

Russ Jordan

I would like to thank the many inspirations in my life, primarily my wife Elizabeth, mother Alicia, and family for encouraging and supporting me in my educational and life pursuits. I would like to also thank my coauthor Charlene Thiessen for the opportunity to work with her in this collaborative work experience and for her professional acumen. Special thanks to John Lampignano, Robert Barnhill and Marigold Linton for their mentorship, guidance, insight, and friendship, they have been awe inspiring.

S.K.I.L.L. Checks and Activities

S.K.I.L.L. stands for Student Key Interaction Lesson Log. These checks and activities have been added to the Basic Client Care 2nd edition text to enhance student learning and increase student interactive learning. Students are encouraged to fill in the SKILL checks and complete the end of chapter questions to increase information retention and gain further insight as to the content materials and experiences. The exercises aid in connecting the identification of the materials with real world applications.

Communication

Communication is transmitting information from one person to another. Probably the only way of being entirely sure that a message is communicated completely is through mind reading, but since that isn't an option for most of us, we have to use the imperfect methods of exchanging ideas, such as speaking, writing, and gesturing. We do this to obtain information from others, provide others with information that we have, develop trust with another person, show that we care about the other person, and relieve stress. Communication is a basic human function that allows us to work with others, have our needs fulfilled, and survive in the world.

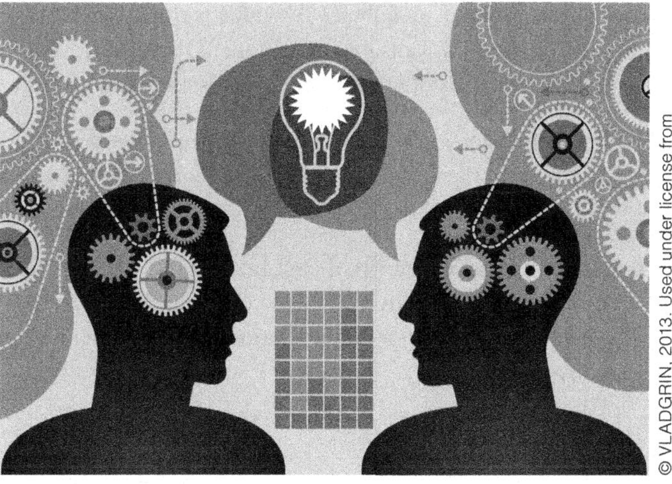

© VLADGRIN, 2013. Used under license from Shuttershock, Inc.

Three Essential Elements of Communication

There are three parts of communication and all must work together for a message to be transmitted correctly.

Sender: The person or group with the information and reason for communicating. This can be an individual, department, or unit of an organization.

Message: The symbols that represent the idea. This may be a verbal message or a nonverbal message and done via face-to-face or another form of transmission. Many times more than one form of transmission is used.

Receiver: The person or group to whom the message is directed. This could be an individual, department, or unit of an organization.

Effectiveness as a Sender

When there is information to be delivered, a way to share that information needs to be found. For example, at the end of a shift, information about the patient needs to be conveyed to the person who will take over the care. The best way to ensure continuity of care is to let the new person know what happened with the patient. For example, if the patient had been to physical therapy and came back within the past 30 minutes, that information should be shared so the patient wouldn't be taken out of the room for walking.

To start the communication process, the sender encodes the message, that is, uses symbols understood by others to deliver the message. This may be by the way of written information, pictures, or even gestures.

One way to ensure that the message sent is the message received is through feedback. When the message is received and decoded, the receiver indicates to the sender what was understood from the message. If the receiver has not correctly interpreted the message, the sender has the opportunity to resend the message in another form that the receiver may better understand.

About 38 percent[1] of human communication is done via speaking. How the words are said influences how the message is received. The combination of intonation, volume, and choice of words is important. A child can be disciplined with a stern look and saying their name in a disappointed tone. Displeasure about a child's behavior can be communicated not only with words but with the way the words are used.

Body language is also an important part of human communication. This includes facial expressions, eye contact, body position, stance, and/or motion. About 55 percent[2] of our communication is done through body language.

Another aspect of communication must be discussed and that is nonverbal communication. At times there are "words-only" communications, like a letter or a class lesson delivered via a computer. However, these are not the most common ways to communicate. And these one-way communications have a higher chance of being incorrectly interpreted due to lack of feedback.

Effectiveness as a Receiver

To effectively send the message, the sender must encode the message in a way that is decodable by the receiver. The receiver must make sure that he or she has decoded the information in a way that matches the speaker's information.

Much like a receiver in a football game, the recipient of the information needs to be at the right place and right time to effectively obtain the information being shared by another healthcare member. When on the receiving end, listening to what the person says takes work. It is easy to become distracted by other people,

---

[1] www.minoritycareernet.com/newsltrs/95q3nonver.html
[2] www.minoritycareernet.com/newsltrs/95q3nonver.html

noises from computers, ringing phones, etc. However, to accurately receive the information, you (the receiver) must pay attention to the sender. Be sure to listen to what the speaker is saying before evaluating it. Don't jump to conclusions before the sender is finished with his or her communication to you. Never assume that what that person is sharing about a patient is something that has been shared before with you. Every situation is different and will not always have the same result.

To assure you've understood the information correctly, paraphrase the message back to the sender. If you do not understand something, ask for clarification. Not understanding the message can harm the patient.

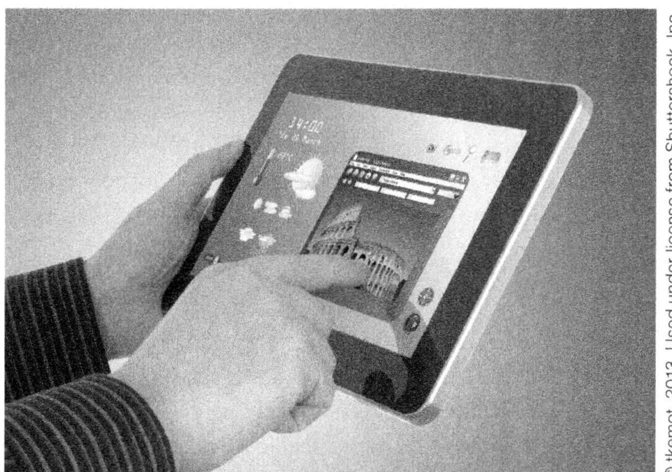

© tkemot, 2013. Used under license from Shuttershock, Inc.

Listening[3]

Throughout a communication engagement, the roles of sender and receiver may be exchanged, modified, or suspended dependent on the type of engagement. Listening is considered a primary factor throughout communication and the degree in which it is engaged is dependent on role, interest, and circumstance of the participant. Listening has several degrees of intensity and has different contexts in which it can be used. Take into consideration the following examples. The reader is listening to the intent or the writer's voice to the degree of reader's comprehension and the writer's ability to convey the information. When observing a scene, the watcher engages in listening behavior within the scope of the viewer's perceptions and ability to interpret the circumstance. Perception of the content is also influenced by the listener, being dependent upon the degree of attention and engagement of the participants; whether their participation is active, passive, or incidental. Listening can be a very engaging and energy consuming process depending on the participants' ability, activity, intensity, and engagement quality.

Considering that a primary portion of what we do in healthcare is communication with the client, it is essential to receive the correct information. This is to form and establish an environment of mutual respectful communication. Creating a forum in which the client is assured of our professionalism, support, and genuine concern of their need, while establishing and strengthening a bond of trust.

---

[3] Jordan, R. (2013). *Basic Client Care: Professional Communications* [PowerPoint presentation and Lecture, Fall, 2013]

Active listening aids in providing and supporting the client's need to be clearly understood and is important in the mission of providing quality client care. It is equally important to distinguish the differences between hearing and listening in reference to communication. The difference between hearing and listening can be demonstrated in the following examples. Hearing is superficial in that it lacks the in-depth experience of engagement and reciprocation of communication cues. For the purposes of this demonstration, it is represented as a two dimensional shape, a circle. Whereas listening, and particularly active listening, is an engagement between the participants of the communication that enlists their participation and interaction at chosen or designated moments during the engagement and so, for demonstration purposes we will represent it as a sphere—a three dimensional object. They both may share some similar basic qualities though the two are still very different.

Looking at humans as a species, we are tailored and designed for face-to-face or in-person communication. When in person, our primary tools for communications; voice, tone, pitch, gestures, facial cues, body posture, listening presence, and interactions are in their dominant forum for optimal performance. This does not prohibit us from expanding on and varying our forms of communication (voice messaging, text, Instagram, Notes, etc.). These expansions of communication formats increase the opportunities for miscommunications due to the fact that the best circumstances for our natural communication may not be present. With each of our primary tools not aligned or accessible for the reciprocation of information (Message) the increased chance for miscommunication rises.

This can be demonstrated in a basic common example. A book is something that we all can identify with, but upon closer examination, we can actually call it a communication. We can break it down in the following way; where the writer is the sender, the book is the message, and the reader is the receiver. The book/message is not able to evaluate or distinguish that the reader/receiver is not receiving its content/message in the context of which the writer/sender had fully intended. If the reader is unable to understand any portion, the book does not know the difference, no matter how puzzled the reader may look.

Consider the differences and essential points between Active Listening and Hearing. When engaging with clients in a healthcare setting which would be considered favorable for gathering information for client intake, learning the client's chief complaint, understanding how their treatment is proceeding, or their concerns. Imagine now that you or your close family member are the client and ask how you would want your practitioner to be according to the following provided examples.

Active Listening Qualities

- In-depth requires more attention and energy

- Provides details increases the opportunity to notice nuances

- Paraphrasing may be utilized to clarify information and for receiver comprehension

- Receiver may use nonverbal skills to enhance more effective communication

- Confers speaker confidence in the receiver and establishes a basis of trust to further engage

Hearing Qualities

- Superficial momentary and inconsistent focused attention

- Catches main subject and familiar generalizations, missing the details

- Uses generalizations and assumptions to fill in the blanks of the communications

How many times have we been witness to or participated in a discussion where one or more participants had different levels of engagement? In discussing with a group, those not directly feeling engaged due to preoccupation, differences, side conversations, or situational distractions may not fully participate or listen. They are hearing what is going on and their attention is elsewhere. This is an example of hearing versus listening.

Factors in Listening[4]

An activity that involves four essential elements represented in Perception, Interpretation, Evaluation, and Action. A healthcare practitioner primarily uses these factors in providing quality care when attentively listening in a conversation to improve their ability to comprehend and respond to a client's message.

The following factors of listening are represented continuously in the professional healthcare field. This configuration of Perception, Interpretation, Evaluation, and Action are repeated in the cycle of communication with a client, peer, administration, and in professional interactions. Based on the healthcare professional's practiced ability, performance and results of these listening factors does their reputation, trust, and credibility increase or decrease? Plain and simple; how well do they listen and provide the level of service expected of them? These are the primary factors of listening, their defining descriptions in their relation to client care.

1. Perception: Recognition and interpretation of information provided through sensory stimuli, memory, insight, intuition, or knowledge gained through experience.
2. Interpretation: A personal understanding or particular view of the information at hand based on personal experience, knowledge, or ideals.
3. Evaluation: The making of an assessment, judgment, and or determination about the significance, value, and condition of an individual(s), object, and or situation. This usually entails a careful study of the relevant influences involved.
4. Action: The process of accomplishing an objective or organized aim, possibly over a period of time, in stages, conceivably requiring additional effort.

Electronic and Telephonic Communication

Computers are used in healthcare daily. Information is input via the keyboard, bar code reader, and/or mouse to request all kinds of information such as diagnostic and treatment orders, patient admission information, or supply inventory. Information is retrieved regarding patient information, test results, etc. The hospital may not allow access to the Internet from inside the hospital to protect the confidentiality of the patient information stored on the computers.

---

[4] Jordan, R. (2013). *Basic Client Care: Professional Communications* [PowerPoint presentation and Lecture, Fall, 2013]

Telephones are ubiquitous: they are in every patient room, on every employee desk, and in every staff member's pocket. Observe these basic etiquette rules when using the phone.

When answering the phone at work (hospital, clinic, doctor's office, etc.):
1. Answer promptly.
2. Identify the facility and your name. In a hospital, identify the unit or floor.
3. Speak clearly and distinctly (do not' eat when answering the phone).
4. Give the caller your undivided attention.
5. Always be courteous, even when the caller is not.
6. If information is requested that isn't readily available, let the caller know that when the information is obtained, it will be given immediately. Then do it.

When answering the phone and taking messages for other people:
1. Make sure the message is given to the correct person (write their name on it).
2. Write down the caller's name, date, time of the call, and the caller's phone number.
3. Include the complete message from the caller.
4. Sign the message slip/email in case there are questions.

If you must put the caller on hold, don't leave them on hold for more than 1–2 minutes. If what the caller needs cannot be found or the person the caller wants to speak to isn't available, take a message and return the call as soon as possible.

When placing a call from work to another place, such as a doctor's office or lab looking for patient test results or to an insurance company to obtain patient coverage information, be sure you have the following before placing the call.
1. Have the patient chart available if necessary.
2. When making a call at someone else's request, write down the information about the call to make sure you have complete and correct information.
3. Get the name of the person who answered the call.
4. Write down all the information obtained, date and time it was obtained, and who gave you the information requested or to whom you gave the information.

Sometimes you'll receive a call from an angry person. Remember, this person is angry about a circumstance that they feel is out of their control. They are not angry with you, so stay calm.
1. Don't put the caller on hold.
2. Listen to what the caller is saying, write it down, and acknowledge his or her anger.
3. Don't allow the caller to become abusive. If that occurs, tell the caller that a discussion of the situation will occur when it can be done without abusive language. If the abuse continues, let him or her know the call will be terminated. Then hang up.

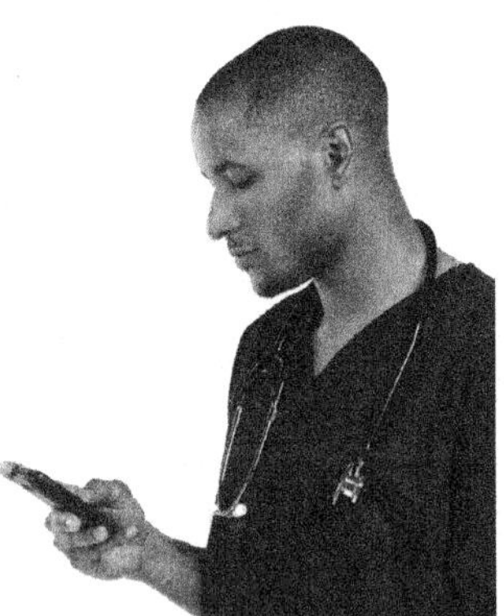

---

[3] C. Thiessen. *Communication and Teamwork in Health Care Organizations.* Retrieved from lecture notes online site: https://maricopa.instructure.com/courses/690855/wiki/culture-and-communication?module_item_id=4354477

[4] www.ojp.usdoj.gov/BJA/evaluation/glossary/glossary_c.htm

4. Document what occurred and give the information to your supervisor.
5. If you are the person in charge, investigate what the person is saying and make changes if possible. Sometimes a situation cannot be changed, in which case you must convey that information to the caller diplomatically.

Cellphones have become the phone of choice for many people and are used everywhere. Healthcare workers use cell phones to communicate with the nursing station and obtain information about their patients. Cellphones need to be used in a considerate manner. When with a patient, set the phone to vibrate mode so you're not interrupted. When using a cellphone and sharing confidential information, be aware of who is within hearing distance.

Healthcare workers use fax machines to send information between units/ floors in a hospital and from hospitals to insurance companies, doctor's offices, etc. Because the information sent over the fax (telephone) lines is confidential and the lines are not secure, care must be taken to ensure that the phone number used is correct. One way to do this is to call the receiver of the information to confirm the fax number.

Email is also used daily in healthcare settings. Again, the confidentiality of information shared via email must be protected. If patient information is sent via email, it must be encrypted so if it goes to the wrong email inbox, it won't be readable. All emails including patient information should include a paragraph at the end that reads something like this:

> This email contains PRIVILEGED and CONFIDENTIAL information intended only for the use of the addressee(s) named above. If you are not the intended recipient of this email or an authorized employee or agent responsible for delivering it to the intended recipient, you are hereby notified that any dissemination or copying of this email is strictly prohibited. If you have received this email in error, please notify us by reply email and delete this email. Thank you for your cooperation.

The notice may not make the information secure, but the recipient will know the information in the email is confidential.

Where Non-Face-to-Face Communication May Fall Short

- When the written language is not the reader's native language.

- When the language does not translate clearly.

- When there is not another word or phrase that properly represents the sender's idea. We've all heard of Shakespeare and his writings, for most persons today, Shakespeare in its original context may require a translator. The terms have changed over the years, but it is still considered English.

- When the words do not have the same meaning; or when the sender and the receiver must agree on a basic definition of the words in context.

- When the sender's facial expressions, emotions, gestures, posture, or intensity/urgency cannot be seen. These are essential cues that are utilized by both the sender and receiver effectively in person-to-person communications to covey particular information.

- Where there are no visual aids to emphasize the communique effectiveness, unless there are illustrations.

- Where there is little to no feedback.

Communicating with Coworkers

First, determine who will receive the information as you may choose to present differently to different people. For example, when dealing with a nurse, information that pertains to the patient's status is most important. When speaking with a physical therapist, the patient's overall status is important, but information about patient's movements may be more important.

When talking with a person outside the hospital, you probably must withhold some information. Make sure the person from outside the hospital/clinic has the proper authorization to receive information on the patient before sharing it.

Next, decide how the information should be shared. When verbally reporting on a patient, be sure you use the correct terms. Be sure you provide the correct times that events occurred as those may be important in further care. When sharing information in a written manner, such as an electronic record, make sure you spell all the words correctly so the reader doesn't have to work to decipher your message.

Speaking with other members of the healthcare team is usually on a peer-to-peer level. A nurse takes care of the overall wellbeing of a patient, and the other team professionals take care of the patient within the scope of their own specialties. All the team members, including the attending physician, are on equal footing and should all have the same goal—taking the best possible care of the patient.

Communicating with Patients

When communicating with patients, remember that they are in an uncomfortable and unknown place. They may be in pain and interacting with people who are alien to their normal life. Express empathy for their feelings and use words that demonstrate an understanding of their discomfort and fears.

Each time you enter a patient's room, follow these steps:
1. Tell the patient in words he or she can understand who you are, what action you will take and why you will do it, when it will happen, and how you will do it. For example, you are going to see a patient to perform vital signs. When you enter the room say, "Hello, my name is Kristine. I am the PCT working on this floor. I will be taking your pulse, temperature, blood pressure, and oxygen level. Your doctor needs to know how you are recovering

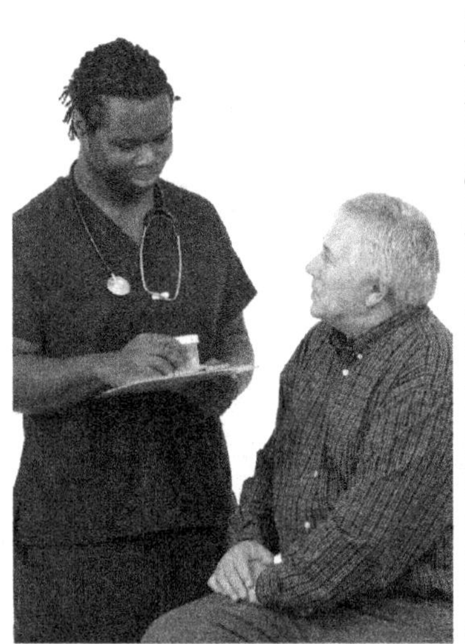

from your surgery. I'll be using the thermometer, blood pressure cuff, and a pulse oximeter, which is a small machine that measures how much oxygen is in your blood."

2. Speak in a normal tone of voice and use common words that the patient can understand. Don't use jargon with a patient. For example, when entering a patient room to obtain a blood pressure, pulse, and temperature, don't talk about "BP, temp, and oxygen sat." The patient won't be able to relate to those terms.

3. Let the patient know that pain or fright or confusion is normal for his or her situation. When a patient knows his feeling are normal, he should relax a little and make his care easier. Let the patient know that if anything you do is uncomfortable, he should speak up immediately so the procedure can be modified to eliminate the discomfort. Always remember: The reason for working in healthcare is to make patients feel better. How information is communicated should always be done in such a way that the patient knows he is important.

Communicating with Family and Friends[5]

S.K.I.L.L. Check

Provide two examples for each consideration.

Cultural Diversity

____
____

Cultural Assimilation

____
____

Acculturation

____
____

Bias

____
____

Notes:

Clients, a majority of the time, arrive at the hospital with family or concerned friends. As professional healthcare practitioners, our primary concerns are the health, wellbeing, safety, and recovery of the client. Considering the circumstance, we the practitioners and the client's present condition are the newly added factors in the equation of the client's life. Certainly it could be said that the attending family and or friends have the very same concerns and deeper emotional investment for their family or friend whom we are providing care for.

Family and friends, out of concern, will offer to assist, provide information, and disclose pertinent and non-pertinent information in an attempt to be helpful. Be aware that they may be able to provide some detailed and important information. Where they can be of assistance and within the professional bounds, allow them to do so. Remember that they are part of the client's support system, which will aid them in recovering. A confrontation between a provider and a family member and or close friend may compromise the stability or wellbeing of a client in distress.

Providing basic support when appropriate can make a difference in comfort, care, mental outlook, cooperation, recovery, and overall experience in the healthcare setting. Practice patience and empathy for the family and friends in the short and long run. Provide a professional standard of care that you would want your family or loved one to receive. A solid standard of quality care creates a positive, supportive, healthy, nurturing, and professional relationship for everyone involved.

Obviously, we as practitioners are required to act within our professional roles and guard the privacy of the client. Allow the practitioners whose scope entails providing the family and or legal designated contact with medical, clinical, and diagnosis information to convey it in their appropriate timeframe and forum. If there is a questionable request of the family or

---

[5] Jordan, R. (2013). *Basic Client Care: Professional Communications* [PowerPoint presentation and Lecture, Fall, 2013]

friends, direct them to an appropriate resource. In the event that there is no resource available at the time, let them know that their questions or concerns will be made known to someone who will be able to assist them and follow through with the communication.

Cultural Considerations[6]

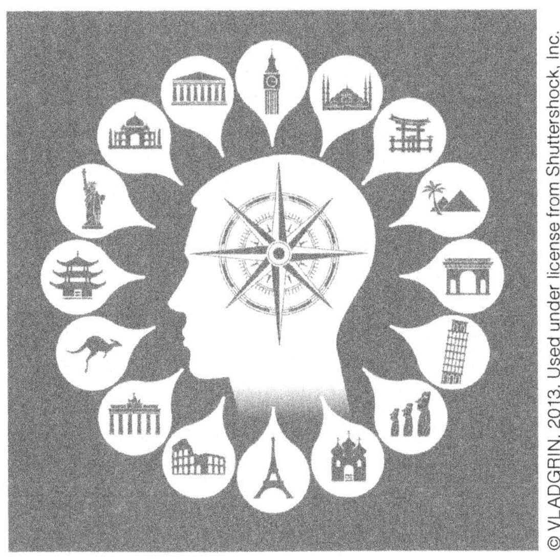

First of all, we to understand what culture means. A good definition comes from the U.S. Dept. of Justice on their Center for Program Evaluation website. Culture is defined as the "shared values, traditions, norms, customs, arts, history, institutions, and experience of a group of people. The group may be identified by race, age, ethnicity, language, national origin, religion, or other social categories or groupings."[7]

All cultures have four basic characteristics:
1. Culture is learned: As children, we learn how to be accepted in our social units and fit into the culture that surrounds us.
2. Culture is shared: A culture shares common beliefs and practices.
3. Culture is social in nature: The shared values develop traditions that are passed down from one generation to the next.
4. Culture is dynamic and constantly changing: As the members of a group change, so does its culture.

Cultural diversity is the variety of human cultures in a specific region, the mixture of individuals and groups with varying backgrounds, experiences, styles, perceptions, values, and beliefs. Traditions play a large part in developing diversity among cultures.

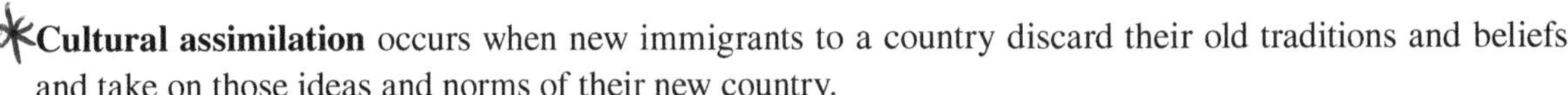

Cultural assimilation occurs when new immigrants to a country discard their old traditions and beliefs and take on those ideas and norms of their new country.

Acculturation is the process by which a culture absorbs the customs of another culture with which it is in direct contact. This occurs when the second- and third-generation members of one culture adopt more of the American (for example) way of life, becoming "Americanized." However, the same people in a culture who have adopted many American ideas may still hold to their traditional ideas in some areas. Acculturation is a slow process and it may take generations to make changes in some traditions.

Bias is any factor that distorts the true nature of an event or observation. For example, a mother watching her daughter perform in a first-grade play at school may think her child shows great acting ability, but it may not be apparent to anyone else. The mother sees her child as talented and gifted, just because it is her child.

Prejudice is the process of pre-judging something. In general, it implies a judgment or opinion on a subject before learning all the facts. Usually, a prejudice is founded on suspicion, intolerance, and the irrational dislike or hatred of other ideas, races, religions, creeds, or nationalities.

---

[6] Thiessen, C. Communication and Teamwork in Health Care Organizations [Word document]. Retrieved from lecture notes online site: https://maricopa.instructure.com/courses/690855/wiki/culture-and-communication?module_item_id=4354477

[7] http://www.ojp.usdoj.gov/BJA/evaluation/glossary/glossary_c.htm

Stereotyping occurs when an oversimplified image of a particular group of people is defined, usually by assuming that all members of the group are alike. For example, someone might state that "all American Indians live in hogans." This may be true of some members of the Navajo culture, but not of all American Indians.

Generalization is a statement that is true about many instances. This is a broad statement or belief based on a limited number of facts, for example, the beliefs, values, behaviors, etc., of a particular group. Knowing that not all information has been obtained should be taken into consideration when applying a generalization to a particular situation.

Discrimination is an act resulting from a particular mindset or prejudice; a way of treating people negatively because of their group identity. Discrimination may be based on age, ancestry, gender, language, race, religion, political beliefs, sexual orientation, family status, physical or mental disability, appearance, or economic status. Acts of discrimination hurt, humiliate, and isolate the victim(s).

What does knowing about different cultures have to do with communication, and then, what does that knowledge have to do with healthcare? Because people who identify with a certain culture develop their ways of communication according to the standards of that group, and not everyone communicates in the same fashion. Immigrants to the U.S., for example, will probably follow the culture of their homeland closely, while second- and third-generation members of the same culture may have incorporated many U.S. attitudes and communication skills. When you encounter people from a different background and culture than your own, you must be aware there will probably be communication difference that could interfere with providing proper medical care.

To develop intercultural communication, first you need to be aware of your own culture, biases, prejudices, and stereotyping. We all have some built-in biases and prejudices toward certain groups of people largely based on how we were raised. When we recognize these biases and prejudices, we can acknowledge that we have these feelings, we can work on not demonstrating them or discriminating against our patient.

Eye Contact

In some cultures, it is considered improper to look directly at a person of authority. These patients may never look at you when you are explaining something. You may consider this a barrier to your communication, but if the patient can paraphrase what has been explained, it was understood.

Touching and Personal Space

Some cultures are comfortable with close physical contact; some are not. If a patient comes from a culture where it is not okay to touch another person or for a male to touch a female, performing some basic patient care functions may be difficult. For example, to take a patient's blood pressure, the arm must be touched and palpated. If a male nurse comes into the room of a Muslim female patient and just starts to unwrap the blood pressure cuff and move toward the patient, the patient may recoil and refuse to allow the procedure to be done. It is necessary to explain what needs to be done, why it needs to be done, and how it needs to be done. At times a patient may verbally agree to a procedure, but still tense up when her personal space is invaded. The healthcare worker needs to be aware of this and do his best to comfort the patient. It may be beneficial to have a member of the patient's family in the room when a procedure needs to be done that the patient finds invasive, even if it is only taking a temperature and pulse.

Language

Although English is the dominant language of this country, according to the U.S. Census Bureau, based on the 2000 census, almost 20 percent of the population under the age of 65 speaks another language at home.[8] There may be a definite lack of communication with a patient because of the language difference. If you encounter a patient who doesn't speak English or not enough English to allow good communication of medical facts, it is important to speak slowly (not loudly; they can hear, just not understand), use simple words and gestures or pictures, and use nonverbal communication (smiling helps alleviate tension). If you work with patients who typically speak another language at home, such as Spanish, it is a good idea to learn some basic sentences in that language, such as "Where does it hurt?" and "How to you feel?" If the patient realizes you are trying to communicate, your efforts will go a long way in establishing a good foundation of trust. If a family member is present who can translate, by all means use him or her to provide information to the patient. If you work in a hospital or large clinic, there may be people on staff who can interpret.

Gestures

Each culture has its own set of gestures to convey feelings. In the U.S., nodding the head up and down indicates yes and shaking the head from side to side means *no*. However, the exact opposite is true in India. If you have a patient from India and he nods his head, you may assume he understands and agrees with what you are telling them, but in reality, he may be saying no. If you notice a that patient appears uncomfortable with a certain gesture you use, you may want to ask what that means to him and explain what you meant when you used it.

Healthcare Beliefs

All cultures respond differently to healthcare. In the U.S., most people feel comfortable being involved in their healthcare, asking the doctor questions, and making their own decisions. However, other cultures have basic healthcare systems based on generations of traditions. A culture may have a strong belief in herbal remedies or religious rites, and if these are not provided, a patient of that culture may not heal well. The following is a list of some basic healthcare beliefs based on different cultures:

---

[8] factfinder2.census.gov/faces/tableservices/jsf/pages/productview.xhtml?pid=ACS_11_5YR_S1601&prodType=table

Table 1.1

Culture	Health Belief	Health Practices	Responses to Pain
Asian American	Health is a balance between energy forces: *yin* (cold) and *yang* (hot). Illness occurs when this balance is disrupted.	They use herbal remedies, acupuncture, acupressure, and foods to restore the balance.	Pain is to be endured; displaying pain in public is disgraceful. These patients may refuse pain medications.
African-American	Supernatural forces can cause illness and influence recovery. Illness may be punishment from God.	They restore harmony by use of prayer, herbs, religious rituals, charms, and amulets.	Tolerating pain is a sign of strength; some may express their pain.
Hispanic/Latino American	Health is a reward from God, it's good luck. Illness may be seen as punishment from God or an imbalance between hot and cold forces.	They use prayers, religious rituals, herbal remedies, and hot and cold remedies to restore balance.	Many will express pain verbally and accept treatment; others may feel pain is to be endured.
American Indian	Health is harmony between man and nature; balance of mind, body and spirit. Illness occurs when this balance is disrupted.	They use rituals; prayer; medication; or plants and herbs to restore harmony. Medicine men may be consulted.	Pain is a normal part of life; tolerating pain means strength.
Middle Eastern	Health is due to spiritual causes. Illness is a punishment for sins. Men make all the medical decisions.	They use meditation, charms, medication, and surgery.	Tolerating pain is a sign of strength; self-inflicted pain is a sign of grief.
Anglo-American	Health is a result of good diet, exercise, and immunizations. Illness is caused by germs, pollutants, etc.	They use home remedies and self-care for minor illnesses; medication and surgery for major illnesses. Diet and exercise are important.	Some will express pain freely; others are more controlled. Pain is alleviated by medications.

As you can see, different cultures approach healthcare with different beliefs. However, remember that not everyone who is a part of a certain culture will hold the same beliefs.

Probably the best way to deal with cultural diversity is to listen to the patient. Asking the patient how he or she wants to be treated gives the patient permission to say no to anything that is uncomfortable.

Communication is a skill that is expected of all healthcare workers. While this may not be listed as part of the job requirements, effective communication is something that must be demonstrated to be considered an exemplary employee.

SKILL Check Activity

Work Place 1

The following is an example of how this would be seen in the workplace setting: A client who arrived twenty minutes before their appointment has been waiting over thirty minutes for their now past appointment time. The client comes to the window and asks the healthcare practitioner how much longer their wait will be. They state that they were on time, followed the examination preparation instructions, and have to go from here to pick up their child. They express how they do not have the time to come again and just sit and wait.

The practitioner knows that the clients' appointments have been delayed due to an emergency response in room 12B where another client has had a heart attack. Most of the situation there is now under control and the required personnel for the frustrated client's exam were involved in handling the emergency situation. The practitioner also understands that the client will not be seen for an additional thirty to forty minutes. The client is obviously upset by the delay and concerned about maybe being rescheduled, having to return, and possibly being late to pick up their child.

Point of Fact

In the scenario of "Work Place 1" please provide a minimum of two examples for each of the following listening factors that are observed. When you have completed them, discuss them with your team members. Explain why you selected the points that you wrote down. In the last portion labeled "Solution", provide your explanation of what and how you would handle the client situation in this scenario. Describe also how you could help repair trust with the client.

- Perception:

    i.

    ii.

- Interpretation:

    i.

    ii.

- Evaluation:

    i.

    ii.

- Action:

    i.

    ii.

Solution: ____

____

____

The situation as presented in "Work Place 1" can be common in various healthcare settings and invariably can cause larger issues if not handled with care and professionalism. The key factors of listening are very important to the practitioner, to come to a satisfactory resolution of this client's needs and care.

In listening, it is essential that the practitioner perceive and acknowledge the client's expressed concerns. The client is particularly interested that the practitioner has gotten what they consider to be the main point of their communication (*Perception*). In this instance, the client would like the practitioner to empathize with their situation and recognize their distress, of which—through no fault of the client—they are now in (*Interpretation*). The practitioner has information in which some they can share and some they cannot. Some of the information to be considered is an explanation to the client, but nothing involving the disclosure of other confidential or private information. Understanding and estimating how long it will take to continue setting up for the client's exam—with patient preparation, personnel, equipment, and supplies are additional factors to consider. The consideration of time—whether or not there is time to properly complete the examination without having to reschedule. Then there is the challenge of making acceptable decisions on each of the aforementioned portions of information, creating an acceptable resolution for the client and the facility, and how to successfully present it to the client (*Evaluation*). Ultimately, all of the above can be considered preparation and eventually, its culmination is dependent upon the last portion "Action". Without successful action or in this instance, a resolution that is acceptable to the client and the facility; this situation could escalate. Simply the client wants to see this situation resolved, handled, and preferably in a solution that satisfies their needs (*Action*).

Throughout the various stages, the practitioner can use the situation to repair trust and in providing the client with some appropriate information, acknowledgment of the situation, and a presentation of possible acceptable solutions if they apply to the situation. The practitioner can lay a reinforced foundation for trust with the client when they listen and provide the client with appropriate feedback and possible acceptable actions.

Respectful and Ideal Communication[9]

Upon initial thought, Respectful and Ideal Communication seem to be synonymous. Considering that most of the time, there is the comingling of various elements from both, there are times when one form may be used to a greater degree than the other. Dependent upon a situation, the speaker chooses which form to engage more actively in and to what degree. When a person speaks to their boss/employer they usually choose to move towards a dialogue infused with more respectful communication. Whereas when a person is communicating with a peer or friend, the dialogue trends more towards Ideal Communication. The speaker is more likely to be more concerned with conveying their point than with considering certain rules, courtesies, or boundaries. Both forms of communication can be used to varying degrees within a communication; it is not an either/or situation. Through closer inspection, Respectful and Ideal Communication reveal their differences and their nature. Though both provide a form of communication, they both do not represent the full framework of each other individually. Together they provide the forum of communication that professional healthcare providers require to create a more complete continuum of care.

---

[9] Jordan, R. (2013). *Basic Client Care: Professional Communications* [PowerPoint presentation and Lecture, Fall, 2013]

Ideal Communication

Ideal Communications is the concept of providing the best circumstances in which shared information can be provided and received by the participants of the communication. In providing the best or ideal conditions with the objective of conveying information, the participants increase the opportunity for optimal results through eliminating inhibiting factors that may reduce the efficiency and effectiveness of the communications.

The most common format for Ideal Communications considers the following guidelines for the Sender/Healthcare Practitioner to consider when providing information to the Receiver/Client when creating an optimal communications forum. The practitioner should hold their gaze, this does not mean to stare uncomfortably at the client, but to make eye contact as needed to insure that they are comfortable and understanding the information.

Correct posture and professional attire project a professional attitude to the client that aids in creating an atmosphere of confidence and capability of care. As part of the professional appearance, each healthcare practitioner needs to consider their hygiene. This includes being properly groomed as well as watching not to use colognes or perfumes that are greatly distinguishable. Remember: clients may have allergies, nausea, or conditions that may be aggravated by strong or particular scents.

Considering that a client may already be in an agitated state due to their condition, the healthcare practitioner must reflect on how the client perceives them. Presenting a calm appearance and a moderate vocal tone provides the client with a more soothing engagement and reduces the opportunity of creating undesired agitation or intensity in the situation.

Lastly, consider reducing physical barriers between you and the client if appropriate for the situation. Considering that the client many times feels displaced by being in unfamiliar settings, presented with unknown possible outcomes, and concerned for someone or their own wellbeing. Providing a more approachable venue creates a supportive environment completely around the client and the best opportunity for ideal communication. Listed below are some of the main factors in Ideal Communications:

- Holding Gaze

- Posture erect, not rigid

- Good Hygiene

- Professional attire

- Moderate vocal tone

- No barriers between you and client

- Relaxed appearance

Respectful Communication

In Respectful Communication with clients, the healthcare practitioner demonstrates consideration, understanding, and or appropriate regard for someone due to their value, achievements, importance, admirable qualities, or position—when having a conversation or communicating with them.

Generally, when speaking to others, being courteous and professional is something mandated by personal, organizational, professional, and or ethical standards. Understanding that even the most intense and critical situations mandate that healthcare practitioners maintain their professionalism and a demeanor of calm. This is to ensure an environment of safety, efficiency, and operational order to provide and maintain the highest standard of quality care. When dealing with the documentation, personal information, and hospital logistics, maintaining confidentiality through guarding privacy and avoiding gossip is an essential component of providing the client a secure environment when they may be feeling most exposed or vulnerable.

Through respectful communication we keep the open communication by acknowledging the client and their needs. Through listening to their health concerns and allowing for them to express themselves thoroughly without unnecessary interruptions we can maintain a level of respect and trust in the client provider relationship. Listed below are some of the main factors in Respectful Communication:

- Be Courteous: Please and thank you

- Maintain Professionalism: Project maturity and competence

- Acknowledgement of Persons: Don't ignore people.

- Do Not Interrupt: Finishing others sentences

- Guard Privacy: Yours and the clients.

- Avoid Gossip: Leads to broken trust.

- Show Interest: Listen Genuinely

- Remain Calm: Even with emergencies

SKILL Check Activity

Instructions: From a distance, observe a conversation in person. List the following information. How many persons are involved in the conversation? _____________________ How far apart do they stand from each other? _____________________ How familiar do they seem to each other (circle one); intimate, friends, acquaintances, impersonal, civil, or hostile? What else did you notice? _____________________

____

____

____

____

Chapter 1 *Questions*

1. List and describe the three components of communication.

2. What is *encoding*?

3. A nurse has directed the patient to take one pill with meals. The nurse means one pill three times a day, approximately 4–6 hours apart, with food.

   a. Describe what may happen if the patient incorrectly decodes this message.

   b. Write down the exact words a nurse should use to communicate the instructions to the patient.

4. Why is body language important to know about? How would you describe body language? What should you do when entering a patient's room? Why is this important?

5. What should be done every time you enter a patient's room? Why is this important?

6. Is it appropriate to use a cellphone in a hospital? What should be considered when making a call about a patient?

7. A 68-year-old man from northern Thailand came to the clinic with his grandson, who was his interpreter. The man had symptoms of weakness, increased thirst, increased urination, and fatigue—classic signs of diabetes mellitus. A blood sugar level is usually obtained to confirm the diagnosis. The nurse explained to the patient, through the grandson, that a blood sample was needed. The patient was horrified at the thought and refused to allow the blood to be drawn. The nurse assumed that he was afraid of the needle and tried to comfort him. His grandson said that his grandfather believed that any loss of blood would make him weaker than he already was. The patient continued to refuse to have the blood test and left the clinic untreated. Is there a cultural problem here to explain the patient's reactions? What might have been done to make the patient more comfortable with the examination? Do you think the patient could have been persuaded to have the test? Why or why not?

8. Why is knowing about another culture important in clear communication?

Vital Signs

Vital signs are the parameters we measure on a patient to determine his or her basic state of health. This includes temperature, pulse, respirations, blood pressure, and oxygen saturation. These parameters are monitored to ensure that treatment is adequate and to assess the patient's state of wellness. Normal ranges for these parameters have been established, and the findings for a particular patient are compared with these ranges to assess a patient's level of functioning. "Normal" varies according to the patient's age, sex, weight, exercise tolerance, and level of physical functioning.

According to the National Institutes of Health,[1] normal vital sign ranges for the average, healthy adult while resting are:
    Blood pressure: 90/60 mm/Hg to 120/80 mm/Hg
    Breathing: 12–18 breaths per minute
    Pulse: 60–100 beats per minute
    Temperature: 97.8–99.1 degrees Fahrenheit/Average = 98.6 degrees Fahrenheit

To obtain a patient's vital signs, follow these steps. Before and as you enter the room:
1. Check the patient's chart to ensure that what is to be done is within the patient's plan of treatment.
2. Obtain all the necessary equipment, ensuring that it's functional.
3. Knock on the door and enter the room. Let the patient know who you are and why you are there.

While in the room:
1. Wash your hands, using soap and water or an alcohol-based hand sanitizer.
2. Put on gloves before touching the patient.
3. Check the patient's ID wristband and have the patient repeat his or her name to you.
4. Perform the vital signs procedure(s).
5. Leave the patient comfortable and with the call light button available.
6. Remove the gloves and wash your hands as you leave the room.

After leaving the room immediately document the findings.

---

[1] www.nlm.nih.gov/medlineplus/ency/article/002341.htm

S.K.I.L.L. Check

What is the importance of documenting Vitals?

1. _______________

2. _______________

3. _______________

Notes:

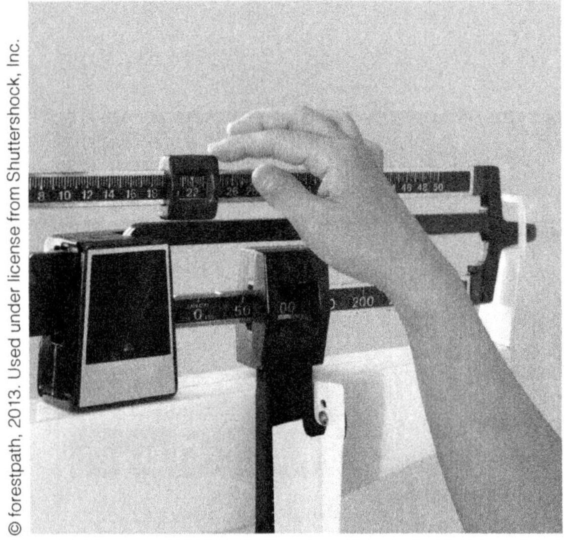

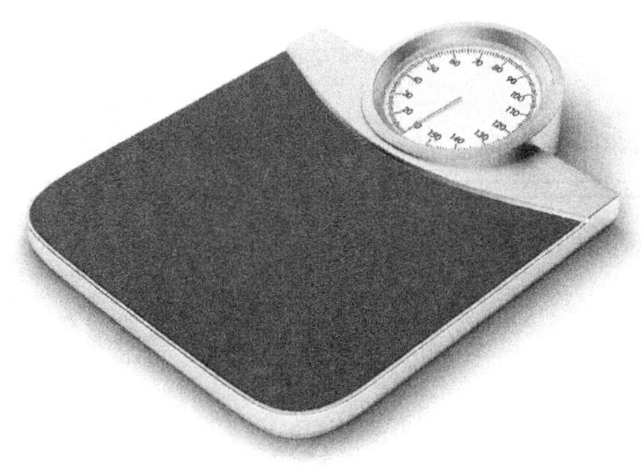

Height and Weight

Height and weight are measured on the first encounter with patients in a clinical setting and may be measured on admission to a hospital. Patients are monitored on an ongoing basis to evaluate their overall health.

Height is measured with a measuring bar, usually attached to the scale. Follow these steps to obtain the height:

1. Raise the measuring bar on the scale and ask the patient to step on the scale, back to the bar. Do this to prevent the patient from stepping into the bar and experiencing an eye or head injury. If the patient faces away from the bar, it's easier for the patient to stand erect.
2. Lower the measuring bar to the top of the patient's head. Record the measurement. If taken in inches, convert an adult's height to feet and inches; leave the height in inches for a child. If the height is taken in centimeters, no conversion is necessary

Weight is obtained on a scale with a balance beam or a digital scale. The balance beam scale must be calibrated before use to assure an accurate weight. To calibrate the scale, place the small and large weights at 0 and be sure the bar floats in the middle of the loop. If it does not float in the middle, adjust the screw until it does.

Follow these steps to obtain a patient's weight on a balance beam scale:

1. Ask the patient to place heavy coats and/or purses and bags on the floor or on a cabinet.
2. Ask the patient to stand on the scale.
3. Adjust the large and small weights along the balance beam until the bar floats in the center of the loop.
4. Record the weight.

To obtain a patient's weight on a digital scale, ask the patient to step on the scale. The weight is automatically displayed.[2]

For patients who are unable to stand, use a sitting scale with a digital scale built into the chair. These are wheelchair-like, with a scale built into the chair. Transfer the patient to the chair, making sure he or she is comfortable. Make sure the patient's feet are on the foot rest, not the floor. Record the patient's weight.

Use a platform scale to weigh patients who are confined to wheelchairs. This type of scale permits the wheelchair to be rolled onto the scale and securely locked in place to obtain the weight. To get an accurate patient weight, the weight of the wheelchair must be subtracted from the total weight.

Patients can also be weighed in a sling lift, which looks like a hammock. Place the patient in the stretcher. A hydraulic lift raises the patient and records the weight.

Temperature

There are five places from which to obtain a patient's temperature. These are (1) the armpit (axillary), (2) the tongue (orally), (3) the rectum (rectally), (4) the ear (tympanic), and (5) the skin (skin sensors). Each site needs different equipment to obtain the temperature and gives a different normal range.

Here are some terms related to temperature and their definitions:
> **Core body temperature**: Operating temperature of the deep structures within the body. This includes the liver, heart, and lungs[3]
> **Afebrile**: No fever; normal temperature
> **Febrile**: Fever (*pyrexia*) with oral temperature above 100° Fahrenheit (37.8° Celsius)[4]
>> **Moderate fever**: Oral temperature of 100–103° Fahrenheit (37.8–39.5° Celsius)
>> **Hyperthermia**: Very high fever, oral temperature greater than 103° Fahrenheit (39.5° Celsius)
> **Hypothermia**: Very low temperature; body temperature less than 95° Fahrenheit (35° Celsius)[5]
> **Baseline**: First set of measured temperature

There are four types of thermometers:
1. Mercury-in-glass;
2. Electronic digital;
3. Tympanic; and
4. Skin sensor.

In 1714 Daniel Fahrenheit, a German merchant and glassblower, created a thermometer that used alcohol to measure temperature changes. Fahren-

---

[2] cengagesites.com/academic/assets/sites/3985_Lindh_ch_24.pdf
[3] medical-dictionary.thefreedictionary.com/temperature
[4] medical-dictionary.thefreedictionary.com/fever
[5] medical-dictionary.thefreedictionary.com/hypothermia

heit chose 32° degrees as the freezing point of water and 212° as its boiling point. The scale was divided into 180 degrees. His scale was based on body temperature.[6]

The mercury-in-glass thermometer was developed in in the 1740s by Anders Celsius, a Swedish astronomer. He was interesting in finding a standard measurement for water at a boiling point and a freezing point. Through his experiments, he developed a glass tube with a bulb at the bottom containing mercury. A change in temperature would move the mercury in the tube. Celsius' original range was 0° for boiling water and 100° for freezing water.[7] A year later Jean-Pierre Christin, a French physicist, mathematician, and astronomer inverted the scale so the freezing point was 0° and the boiling point was 100°. He divided the scale in 100 sections and named it *centigrade*.

Today the mercury-in-glass thermometer for human use has been banned by many countries due to mercury's toxicity. The U.S. Environmental Protection Agency recommends that mercury thermometers be removed from all homes.[8]

Electronic digital thermometers were created to measure oral temperatures. These types of thermometers use a thermal resistor to determine the temperature and convert that measurement into a digital format that corresponds to the Fahrenheit and/or Celsius scale.[9] Tympanic thermometers use infrared radiation and a thermopile detector[10] that is inserted into the ear. This type of thermometer records temperature in two seconds, whereas it takes a digital thermometer about 60 seconds to record the temperature.

Tympanic thermometers take a patient's temperature during surgery and are used as a temperature probe for an unconscious patient.[11] Skin sensor thermometers are placed on the skin and record the temperature using an infrared thermographic scanner. These are used on babies in the neonatal intensive care units and can be bought over the counter.

The average normal temperature range depends on age and where on the body the temperature is taken.[12]

Table 2.1

Fahrenheit	0–2 years	3–10 years	11–65 years	> 65 years
Oral	—	95.9–99.5 F 35.5–37.5 C	97.6–99.6 F 36.4–37.5 C	98.2–100.2 F 36.8–37.9 C
Rectal	97.9–100.4 F 36.6–38 C	97.9–100.4 F 36.6–38 C	98.6–100.6 37–38.1 C	97.1–99.2 F 36.1–33.4 C
Axillary	94.5–99.1 F 34.7–37.3 C	96.6–98 F 35.8–36.6 C	95.3–98.4 F 35.2–38.8 C	96–97.4 F 35.5–36.3 C
Tympanic	97.5–100.4 F 36.3–38 C	97–100.0 F 36–37.7 C	96.6–99.7 F 35.9–34.6 C	96.4–99.5 F 35.7–37.5 C
Core	97.5–100 F 36.3–37.7 C	97.5–100 36.3–37.7 C	98.2–100.2 F 36.8–37.9 C	96.6–98.8 F 35.8–37.1 C

[6] inventors.about.com/od/fstartinventions/a/Fahrenheit.htm

[7] www.astro.uu.se/history/celsius_scale.html

[8] yosemite.epa.gov/ochp/ochpweb.nsf/content/heating.htm

[9] ezinearticles.com/?Thermometers—A-History&id=1633430

[10] Electronic devise that converts thermal energy to electronic energy; www.novalynx.com/glossary-t.html

[11] www.ehow.com/how-does_4922559_tympanic-thermometers-work.html

[12] www.minoritycareernet.com/newsltrs/95q3nonver.html

Follow these steps to take a temperature:[13]
1. Determine the appropriate site.
2. Assure that the thermometer is working properly.
3. Insert the probe into the appropriate body site.
4. Leave the probe in place for the recommended time.
5. Check the reading and write it down.

A rectal thermometer gives the most accurate temperature. Follow these steps to obtain a rectal temperature:
1. Ask the patient to lie prone (on the stomach).
2. Lubricate the end of the thermometer probe and anus with petroleum jelly.
3. Insert the thermometer into the anus to a depth of approximately 1 inch.
4. A glass thermometer should be left in place for 2 minutes. A digital electronic thermometer should be left in place for 20 seconds.

An axillary (armpit) thermometer is the least accurate thermometer. Follow these steps to take an axillary temperature:
1. Make sure the armpit is dry.
2. Insert the thermometer into the armpit.
3. Close the armpit by holding the elbow close to the body.
4. Leave the thermometer in place for 4–5 minutes.

Follow these steps to take an oral temperature:
1. Place the thermometer below the tongue toward the back of the mouth.
2. Ask the patient hold the thermometer in place with the lips (not the teeth) and breathe through the nose.
3. Leave thermometer in place 3 minutes.

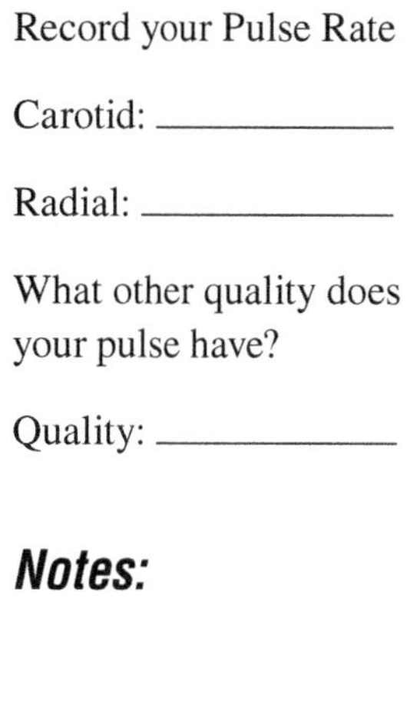

Record your Pulse Rate

Carotid: _______________

Radial: _______________

What other quality does your pulse have?

Quality: _______________

Notes:

Earwax, ear infections, and ear tubes do not interfere with accurate readings from a tympanic (ear) thermometer. Follow these steps to take a tympanic temperature:
1. Pull the ear upward to straighten the ear canal.
2. Aim the tip of the probe midway between the opposite eye and earlobe. Be gentle when inserting the thermometer.
3. Leave in place 2 seconds.

Pulse

Measuring the pulse assesses how fast the heart is beating. The *pulse* is the pressure felt against an artery when the heart beats. The pulse is measured to check how well the heart is working, to find the cause of symptoms like rapid heart rate, dizziness, fainting, shortness of breath,

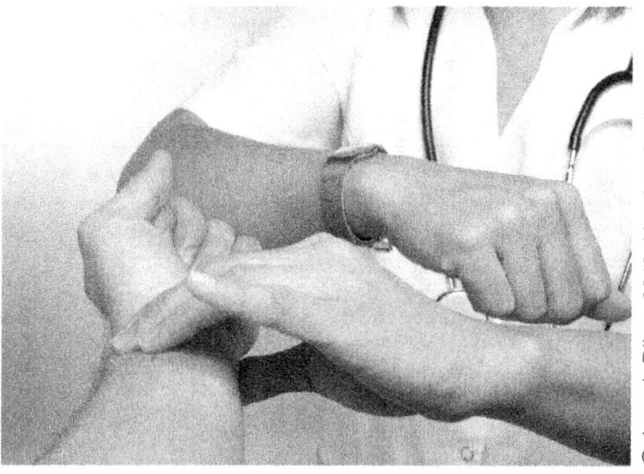

---

[13] Information obtained from www.bannerhealth.com/incfiles/housecalls/peds/FeverInfectionsCrying/FeverHowtoTaketheTemperature.htm

or chest pain, to check on blood flow after an injury, to check on medicines that may cause a slow heart rate, and to check general health level.

Here are some terms related to the pulse:

Rhythm: Regular or irregular
Rate: Speed of the heart rate: slow, average, or fast
Strength: Bounding or thready
Tachycardia: Fast rate (> 100 beats per minute)
Bradycardia: Slow rate (< 60 beats per minute)
Resting heartrate: The pulse taken upon first waking in the morning or after sitting for 10 minutes

The places to take a pulse are:

- **Radial**: Inside of the wrist
- **Apical**: Between the 4th and 5th ribs, over the apex of the heart
- **Carotid**: In the neck below the jawbone, halfway between main neck muscles and windpipe
- **Femoral**: Over the groin
- **Brachial**: Inside the upper arm near the elbow
- **Temporal**: On the temple directly in front of the ear
- **Popliteal**: Behind the knee
- **Dorsalis pedis**: Top of the foot
- **Tibial**: On the medial side of the ankle

Before measuring a pulse, make sure you have a watch with a second hand. Then follow these steps to measure the pulse

1. Use the index and middle finger over the pulse point. (Do not use the thumb as it has a pulse that you can feel.)
2. Press on the pulse point until you can feel the pulsation of the artery. Do not press so hard enough that you obliterate the pulse.
3. Hold your fingers on the pulse and count the number of beats for 30 seconds.
4. Multiply that number by 2 to obtain the beats per minute and write down the number.

The table below shows average pulse rates based on gender and age.[14]

Table 2.2	Resting Heart Rate
Age or Fitness Level	**Beats per Minute (BPM)**
Babies to age 1	100–160
Children ages 1–10	70–120
Children ages 11–17	60–100
Adults	60–100
Well-conditioned athletes	40–60

Circumstances that can affect pulse rates include activity level, ambient temperature, emotions, body size, medication use, and fitness level. A normal adult pulse is about 72 beats per minute, but an athlete's pulse

---

[14] www.nlm.nih.gov/medlineplus/ency/article/003399.htm

rate may be below 50 per minute due to the good condition of the heart muscle with a higher amount of blood pushed through the arteries with each heartbeat.

Respirations

Respirations are measured by the chest rise and fall, or each inspiration and expiration. This is also called the **respiratory cycle. Respiratory rate** can increase with fever and other medical conditions.

Here are some terms related to respirations:
    Rate: Frequency of the respiratory cycle
    Rhythm: Regularity of the respiratory cycle or spacing of the breaths; described as regular or irregular
    Symmetry: The chest wall motion; both sides of the chest should rise and fall at the same time and with the same motion
    Character: A description of the breathing, which can be described as:
        Deep: Characterized by fully filling the lungs; may happen if the patient knows their respiratory rate is being evaluated
        Shallow: Characterized by drawing in minimal air, not fully inflating lungs
        Labored: Characterized by increased effort to inhale; the accessory muscles of respiration are involved; muscles located in the neck and upper chest
        Moist: Characterized by an accumulation of secretions, such as saliva and mucus, collecting in the throat
        Stertorous: Characterized by a heavy snoring or gasping sound

Other terms describe the adventitious sounds heard in conjunction with breathing.
    Adventitious sounds are the additional sounds heard along with the normal breathing sounds (these are heard when using a stethoscope)
    Rales or **crackles**: Intermittent, brief, nonmusical sounds; caused by narrowing of the bronchi due to fluid in the lungs. **Fine crackles** sound like rolling hair between fingers. **Coarse crackles** sound like opening Velcro
    Rhonchi or **wheezes**: Can be heard with inspiration and expiration, are somewhat musical in sound, may be shrill and squeaking or snoring and moaning
    Stridor: A high-pitched harsh sound heard during inspiration
    Rubs: Low-pitched grating, creaking sounds

Here are some terms associated with abnormal breathing patterns:
    Dyspnea: Difficult or labored breathing
    Apnea: Absence of respirations
    Tachypnea: Rapid respiratory rate above 25 rpm
    Bradypnea: Slow respiratory rate, usually below 10 rpm

orthopnia

Orthopnea: Severe dyspnea in which breathing is difficult in any position other than sitting erect or standing

Cheyne-Stokes: Periods of dyspnea followed by periods of apnea, frequently noted in the dying patient

(Chain-stokes)

Measure respirations when you measure the pulse. This is done in conjunction with measuring the pulse. Don't tell the patient about measuring respirations because just knowing that the respirations are being observed will change the pattern. Follow these steps to measure respirations:

1. When you have finished taking the pulse, keep your fingers on pulse.
2. Count how many times patient inhales for 15–30 seconds.
3. Multiply count by 4 (if measured for 15 seconds) or 2 (if measured for 30 seconds).
4. Record the number.

Here are the average resting respiratory rates by age:[15]

Newborn: 44 breaths per minute

Infants: 20–40 breaths per minute

Children (ages 1–7): 18–30 breaths per minute

Adults: 12–20 breaths per minute

Blood Pressure

For patients, blood pressure is probably the most familiar vital sign. Obtaining the **blood pressure** is a way to assess the function of the patient's heart. The pressure measured is that of the blood pushing on the walls of the arteries and veins while moving through the body. The beating heart pushes the blood. A high blood pressure leads to thinning of the blood vessels' walls because of the pressure exerted on them. High blood pressure can result in **aneurysms** (ballooning of the vessel wall) and ruptures. Low blood pressure means that the blood isn't being pushed hard enough to reach the farthest point from the heart effectively. It can lead to fainting and poor perfusion of the extremities. Loss of blood flow to the extremities can result in tissue death.

Here are some terms related to blood pressure:

Systole: Heart muscle contraction; the force required to pump the blood out of the heart into the aorta and the arteries to circulate through the body

Diastole: Heart muscle relaxation; the pressure in the arteries when the heart is at rest

Blood pressure is written as systolic over diastolic; for example: 120/80 mmHg (millimeters of mercury)

Here's a list of some blood pressure devices:

Manual: Measuring blood pressure by human means, using the sphygmomanometer and stethoscope

---

[15] books.google.com/books?id=AUhJKmKJ_eEC&pg=PA573#v=onepage&q&f=false

Digital/electrical: Measuring blood pressure using a device powered by electrical means; a stethoscope is not required

Arterial line: A catheter inserted in the arterial system that measures the pressure inside the arteries

Doppler: An ultrasound system that measures blood flow and blood pressure by bouncing sound waves off circulating red blood cells

Here are the normal blood pressure ranges for adults:

Hypotension: Systolic 90 or below and diastolic 60 or lower

Normal: Systolic below 120; diastolic below 80

Prehypertension: Systolic from 120–139; diastolic from 80–89

Stage 1 hypertension: Systolic from 140–150; diastolic from 90–99

Stage 2 hypertension: Systolic 160 or more; diastolic 100 or more[16]

Hypersensitive Crisis: Systolic 180 or more and diastolic 110 or more

Hypersensitive crisis means that blood pressures in the 180/110 range place the person in a crisis category and immediate medical treatment should be sought out. This is considered to be a critical care matter due to the increased risk of potential stroke, heart attack, and with prolonged exposure permanent damage to the heart.[16]

Table 2.3		
Blood Pressure Category	**Systolic Pressure**	**Diastolic Pressure**
Hypotension	90 lower	60 lower
Normal	120–91	80–61
Prehypertension	120–139	80–89
Hypertension Stage 1	140–159	90–99
Hypertension Stage 2	160 or more	100 +
Hypersensitive Crisis	180 +	110 +

In children, blood pressure varies with age. Here's a rough guide to the average blood pressure in normal children:[17]

Table 2.4							
Age	Birth	6 mo.	1 yr.	2 yr.	6 yr.	8 yr.	10 yr.
Systolic BP	70	90	90	92	95	100	105

Many factors can increase blood pressure. They include:

Table 2.5	
Age	Pain
Disease	Gender
Activity	Obesity
Emotions	Heredity
Stimulants	Medications

---

[16] www.mayoclinic.com/health/blood-pressure/HI00043

[17] medinfo.ufl.edu/year1/bcs/clist/vitals.html#RESP

Many factors can decrease blood pressure such as:

Table 2.6	
Fasting/dieting	Resting/relaxing
Depressants	Weight loss
Medications	Cricial conditions
Postural hypertension (dizziness)	

When taking a blood pressure, these points are key to obtaining a "good" blood reading:
- Correctly palpate the brachial pulse.
- Use a correctly sized cuff (both width and length). If the cuff is too tight, you could get a false high blood pressure. If the cuff is too loose, you could get a false low reading.

Here are some blood pressure "dos":
- The correct patient position is essential. The blood pressure should be taken at chest level. If the arm is higher than chest level, you will get a false low reading. If the arm is lower than the chest, you can get a false high blood pressure.
- If you get an abnormal reading, repeat the blood pressure procedure.

Here's a blood pressure "don't":

Do not take a measurement at an IV site, the site of an arm injury, an **edema** (swelling), or any arm abnormality.

The two pieces of equipment you need to obtain a blood pressure are
a **sphygmomanometer** (the blood pressure cuff) and a stethoscope.

There are different types of sphygmomanometers. The **aneroid** sphygmomanometer, which means the measurement is obtained without the use of fluids, is the most commonly used. The **mercury** sphygmomanometer uses mercury to measure blood pressure. The sphygmomanometers work in a similar manner.

The cuff used in conjunction with the sphygmomanometer comes in different sizes. The size you used must correlate with the girth of the patient's arm. A cuff that's too small will give a false high reading, and a cuff that's too large will give a false low reading. The width of cuff should be approximately 20 percent longer than the diameter of the patient's upper arm. The cuff contains a rubber bladder that fills with air as it is inflated.

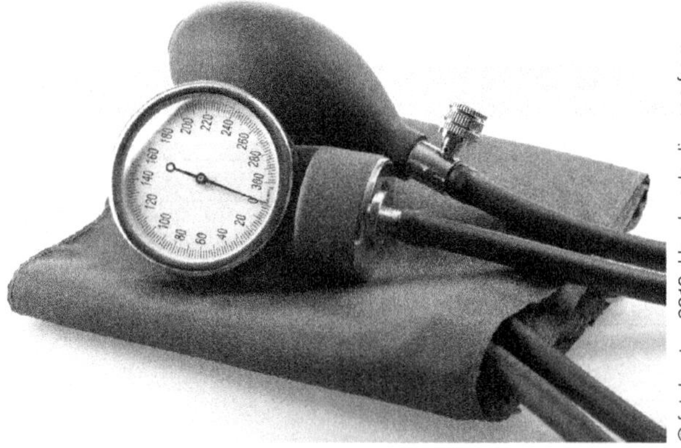

An aneroid sphygmomanometer:
  - doesn't have a mercury column, only a round gauge;
  - is calibrated in millimeters of mercury (mmHg);
  - is lined, with each line on the gauge representing 2 mm of Hg; and
  - should be positioned at eye level for correct readings.

A mercury sphygmomanometer
  - contains a long column of mercury;
  - is lined, with each line on the gauge representing 2mm of Hg;
  - must be placed on a flat, level surface or mounted on a wall or stand; and
  - has a level of mercury that should be at zero when viewed at eye level.[18]

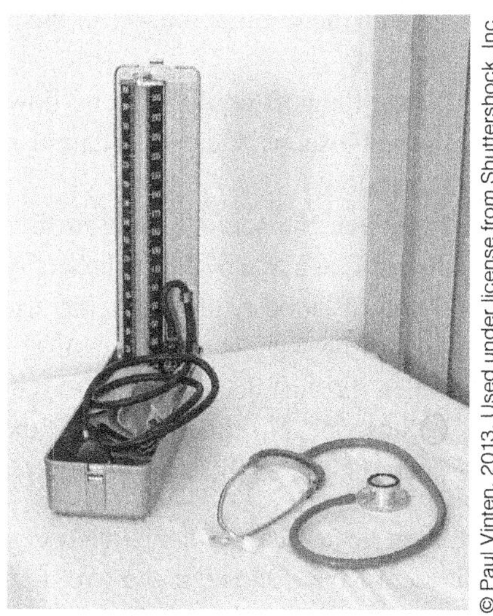

Follow these steps to measure the blood pressure:
  1. Place the edge of the cuff about 1 inch above the bend of the elbow and close the cuff around the arm. The cuff should be on a bare arm and the artery marker should be over the brachial artery. Allow only two fingers to fit under the cuff for a snug fit.
  2. Ask the patient to sit, with the back supported and legs uncrossed. Keep the patient's upper arm at heart level, by supporting the lower arm and keeping the arm still.
  3. Put the stethoscope earpieces in your ears and place the stethoscope bell at the side of the cuff away from the heart and over the brachial artery, found in the inner area of the bent elbow.

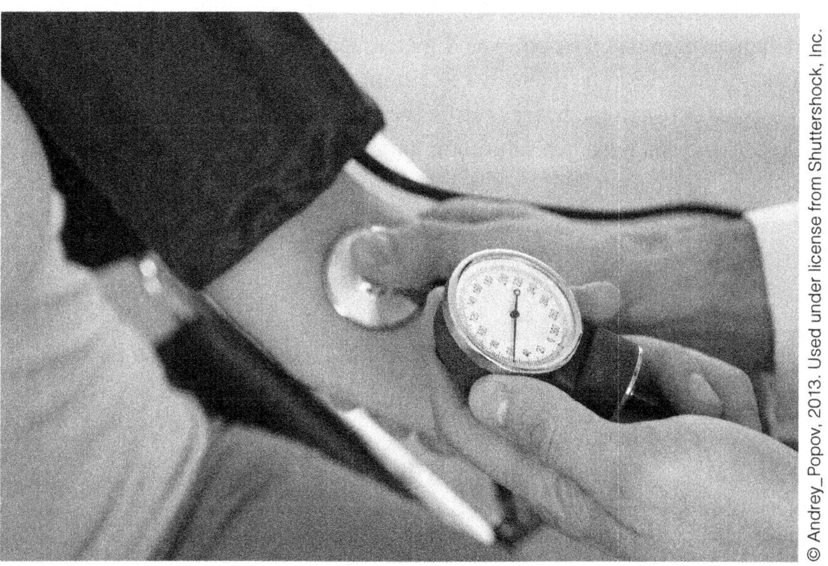

18 Faculty.nwacc.edu/tbriggs/CNA I files/Vital Signs 2.ppt

4. Tighten the screw at the side of the rubber bulb, then squeeze the bulb. Pump air into the bulb to expand the cuff.
5. Inflate the cuff until the blood flow through the brachial artery stops and no sound is heard through the stethoscope. Quickly inflate the cuff to 30 millimeters of mercury (mmHg) above the point of no blood flow.
6. Untighten the screw to loosen the valve in the bulb and lessen the air pressure. The pressure will decrease at a rate of 2 mmHg/sec. As the pressure falls and with your eye on the dial, listen for the first sound of blood returning to the artery. At the first sound, note the location of the needle on the dial. This is the systolic blood pressure.
7. When the cuff decompresses to the point that blood flows freely in the artery, no sound will be in the stethoscope. Note the location of the needle. This is the diastolic blood pressure.
8. Record both numbers immediately.[19, 20]

The American Heart Association recommends taking the patient's blood pressure twice while standing, then record the average of the two; next, take it twice while sitting and record the average of those two. Document which pressure was taken with the patient standing and which was taken when sitting. Use the sitting measurement as your final reading; the standing measurement is for reference only. [21]

Oxygen Saturation

The concentration of oxygen in the blood is measured with a **pulse oximeter**. A pulse oximeter is a small photoelectric device that is placed on the finger or earlobe and measures the pulsations of the capillaries. A beam of red and infrared light passes through the pulsating capillary bed.

Oxygen saturation of the blood is determined by comparing the different colors of blood, where oxygenated blood is brighter red than deoxygenated blood. An oximeter measures the heart beat and notes the intensity of the color between the heart beats. The intensity of color of the both oxygenated and deoxygenated blood minus the intensity of color between the heart beats is the oxygenated blood. This number is displayed on the pulse oximeter screen and is the oxygen saturation, or O2 sat, of the blood.[22]

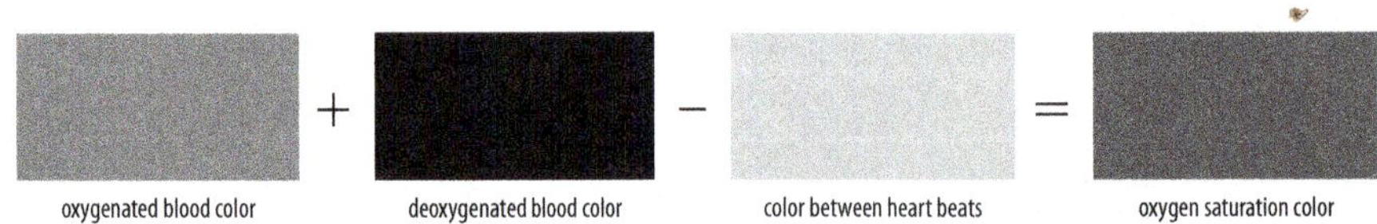

Pulse oximetry devices are
    Portable: Battery-powered devices;
    Electric: Devices that run off electric power and keep digital records of the oxygen saturation; and
    Disposable/nondisposable: Disposable devices are single-use probes attached to an earlobe; nondisposable devices are placed on the finger.

---

[19] www.dummies.com/how-to/content/taking-your-blood-pressure-correctly.html
[20] blog.schoolhealth.com/bid/56713/9-Tips-for-Taking-Accurate-Blood-Pressure-Readings
[21] www.steeles.com/catalog/takingBP.html
[22] http://www.medicinenet.com/oximetry/article.htm

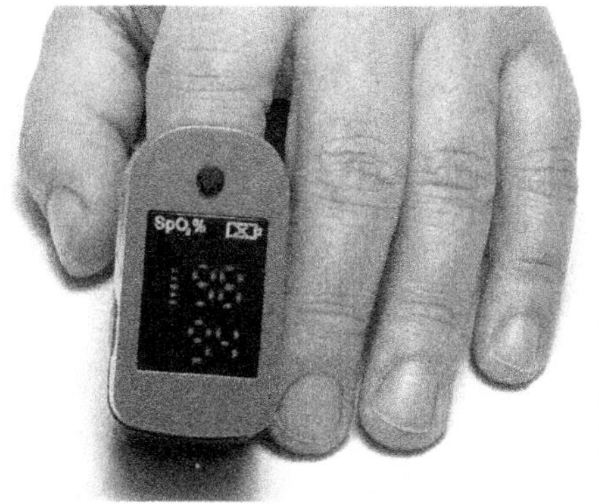

A portable nondisposable pulse oximeter

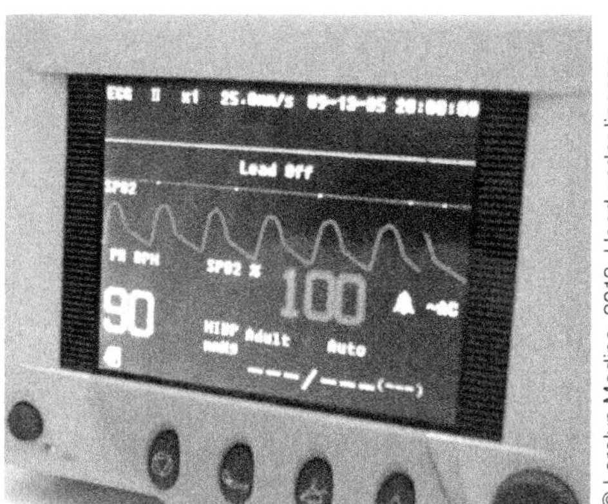

An electric pulse oximeter monitor

The one term related to oxygen saturation that you should know is:
> **Hypoxemia**: Low oxygen level, below 95%

Normal values are in the range of 95–100%.

Abnormal values of
> **Less than 90%**: Oxygen therapy needed
> **Less than 85%**: Critical situation, patient will be taken to the ICU
> **Less than 75%**: Life threatening

Follow these steps to obtain an oxygen saturation level:
1. Remove any nail polish from the **digits** (fingers) where the sensor is to be applied.
2. Turn on the device.
3. Place device on finger. The reading will appear on the screen.

Vital signs are an important factor in patient assessment. Policies and procedures written by individual hospitals/medical clinics should be followed when obtaining vital signs. Always be professional when obtaining vital signs, record them accurately, and report any abnormalities found to the RN or physician caring for the patient.

Blood Glucose Level[23]

Blood Glucose Level is also known as blood sugar level; this reading is the indication of the amount of sugar in the bloodstream. The levels of blood sugar become significant when considering if a person is developing or has developed diabetes. Low or high blood sugar levels may significantly impact the type and course of care. Blood sugar levels are particular concern of individuals with diabetes or a family history of this condition and or disease.

Blood Glucose levels may vary from patient to patient depending on various factors that may include: time of day, dietary habits, last meal eaten, medication, weight, physical inactivity, race, illness and other factors. The following table provides a general view of how blood glucose levels are commonly characterized. Even with this information, any questions or concerns when considering blood glucose levels would best be directed to a physician or qualified specialist.

Table 2.7		
Blood Glucose Level	**Ranges mg/dl**	**Possible Symptoms**
Dangerously low	50-below	Unconsciousness
Low	65-50	Shakes, Hunger
Normal	70-100	None
Elevated	100-125	None
At Risk	126-155	Organ Complications (OC)
High	156-200	Glucose in Urine (OC)
Dangerous	250-above	Altered Mental Function Organ Complication (OC)

Patient Medical History[24]

Pertinent medical information is required to determine the best course of treatment for clients. In order to determine the status of the client, it is imperative that the practitioner obtains the information needed to provide the best treatment available. The patient history or information aids in creating a proper assessment and course of action. This information can be obtained in several formats.

Patient Medical Record

This is a document collection of the patient's past illnesses, treatments, medications, and procedures. These records may or may not be complete depending on various factors; has the patient recently moved, is this the first time at this facility, does the patient have regular checkups, and possibly, are the records from this country. Whether any or all of these could apply to the situation, it is imperative to determine that the records match with the patient before including the information in the patient assessment and treatment.

---

[23] http://www.webmd.com/

[24] Jordan, R. (2013). *Basic Client Care: Client Assessment* [PowerPoint presentation and Lecture, Fall, 2013].

Patient Exchange

Many times the best person to inform the practitioner on the recent and past history of the patient is the client themselves. When it is possible and applicable, confer with the client to determine this valuable information. During the patient triage and intake, listen and review the information ascertained with the client to clarify as much of the present situation as possible. Some examples of questions may be as follows:

- Have you had any recent illnesses or injuries?
- Do you have any known allergies to food, medication, or other?
- Have you had this or something similarly occur previously?
- When was your last visit to the doctor or hospital? What was it for?
- Are you on any prescription medications; if so which ones?
- Are you taking any over the counter medications; if so which ones?
- Have you ever been hospitalized before; if so for what and when?
- Do you have any chronic conditions or illnesses?

In most instances, it has been found to be extremely helpful to just let the client speak about how they feel and about their past health to some degree. Some clients have had injuries or illnesses that they have lived with for an extended period; to them there is nothing special or different about these conditions because they have been a regular part of their lives, sometimes for years or decades. Example: A 47-year-old client has lived with Spina Bifida (a congenital birth defect) for their whole life and may not think to mention the condition. It is not unusual for patients with Spina Bifida to have related conditions: heart problems, bowel or bladder issues, latex allergy sensitivities.

Responsible Family Member/Liaison

Possibly due to circumstances, illness, condition, or special circumstances the patient's records, history, and or information may be provided by another responsible party. This person may be a family member, friend, or official representative. It is important to first determine the role as well as legal documentation (medical power of attorney) when conferring with the patient's respective liaison.

Emergencies

In some instances, there is no opportunity or information to be gathered on a patient due to the circumstances; treatment may have to be provided without even the knowledge of a patient's name. In these occurrences, particular care must be taken in maintaining records for documentation purposes and to later be matched to any existing records if any are discovered.

Exercises

Point of Fact

Select and list three to five of the most important facts about each of the vital signs explained in the text.

Heart Rate:

Oxygen Saturation:

Pulse:

Blood Pressure:

Temperature:

Road Scholar

Divide the class into groups; each group will create a poster that will represent a specific vital sign without using words and only drawing descriptors. (The only written words allowed are those used to identify the heading on the poster paper. Have one member of the group explain the subject to the group present, and then have each group rotate around to the next subject (vital sign). At each rotation, the presenter will select a member of the group to stay and present the material they were just presented to the incoming group. The group may ask the presenter questions on the material. Each member of the group will get a designation (a letter, number, or color) this determines the peer instructor of the subject. No note taking is allowed.

What Happens When?

Using the graphic organizer "What Happens When?" on page 137 consider what happens to the vital signs of a client suffering from a condition, illness, or traumatic event (heart attack, stroke, asthma attack, etc...). In the center triangle place the considered condition and in the additional vital areas review, discuss, and make notes as to what would like likely happen in the event of this condition occurring. Review them in the following order:

1. Respiration;
2. Heart Rate;
3. Blood Pressure

What additional Vital signs changes might be a consideration when providing care for the client and their condition?

____

____

____

Chapter 2 *Questions*

1. Name three factors that might increase a client's blood pressure.

2. When taking a pulse, why would you use the popliteal pulse site instead of the radial pulse site?

3. Which reading—diastolic or systolic—measures the pressure when the ventricles of the heart have relaxed?

4. What is the average pulse range for infants?

5. Name two things you should do immediately upon entering a client's room for the first time.

6. Name four pulse sites.

7. When counting a patient's respirations, what is one thing you should never do?

8. What is *orthopnea*?

9. What could be said about a patient with an oxygen saturation level of 87%?

10. What is pyrexia?

Infection Control

Infection

What is an infection? How does it happen? How can it be stopped? Answers to these questions must be part of the medical professional's awareness when caring for patients.

An **infection** is the invasion of the body by a pathogenic microorganism. **Microorganisms** are single-cell organisms that can only be seen with a microscope. When speaking of microorganisms, the conventional wisdom equates this with bacteria, viruses, and protozoas.

Microorganisms exist in our environment in the air, soil, water, and food. People carry microorganisms with them in the mouth, nose, respiratory tract, gastrointestinal tract, and skin. Other sources of microorganisms are animals, both domesticated and wild, clothing, and furniture. Just being alive constantly exposes people to microorganisms. Microorganisms that reside in our body are called the **normal flora**. More than 200 species of bacteria comprise the normal flora of a human body.[1] Many of these organisms live in one part of the body without deleterious effect, but cause an infection when they move to a different part of the body. For example, *Streptococcus pneumoniae* lives in the upper respiratory tract (nose, throat, and pharynx) without a problem, but if it gets into the lower respiratory tract (trachea, bronchi, and lungs), it causes pneumonia.[2] *Escherichia coli* is a bacterium that lives in the human intestinal tract. As long as the bacteria stay in the intestinal tract, it's not harmful; however, when it moves into the urethra, it causes a urinary tract infection.[3]

Healthy individuals have an immune system that produces specialized cells to destroy pathogenic microorganisms when they enter the body. However, people with a compromised immune system lack adequate defenses to fight off the microorganisms. When a microorganism enters the body, it multiplies, invades structures in the body, and produces disease.

---

[1] textbookofbacteriology.net/normalflora.html

[2] textbookofbacteriology.net/normalflora.html

[3] crohn.ie/archive/primer/normflor.htm

Antibiotics help humans' systems kill the bacteria that cause disease. These include medications such as penicillin and erythromycin and all their derivatives. Over time and exposure to antibiotics, some of the organisms have become resistant to the antibiotics. Two of the common drug-resistant organisms are MRSA (methicillin-resistant *Staphylococcus aureus*) found in the upper airways and VRE (vancomycin-resistant enterococcus) found in the intestines. These types of infections are most often found in hospitals and other healthcare settings. Another bacterium that is becoming drug resistant is tuberculosis. The two medications that historically have been used to kill the *Mycobacterium tuberculosis* bacteria are isoniazid and rifampicin. Some strains of the bacteria have been found to be resistant to these medications.[4]

Viruses are extremely tiny microorganisms, 100 times smaller than a bacterial cell. A bacterial cell is 10 smaller than a human cell, and a human cell is 10 smaller than the diameter of a human hair. Viruses need a host to live. Viruses enter the body from the environment or from other individuals. They go from soil to water to air to humans via nose, mouth, or any breaks in the skin and seek a cell to infect. A virus attaches to the cell and injects its DNA into the cell. The invading DNA takes over the cell and uses its enzymes to make new viral cells. These new viral cells kill the cell they invaded and then when break free and search for new cells to inhabit.[5] The body fights off these viruses by producing antibodies. These antibodies remember the virus and next time that virus invades the body, it's killed immediately.

Vaccination is the method to prevent the spread of viruses. Smallpox is caused by a virus that has been attacked worldwide through systemic vaccination, and in 1980 smallpox was deemed completely eradicated. Antibiotics cannot kill viruses and there are few medications that have been developed that can. Some antiviral medications have been developed to treat HIV (human immunodeficiency virus). They don't kill the HIV virus, but they do keep it from replicating. Tamiflu is another antiviral medication developed to prevent influenza. However, the virus is capable of quickly adapting to the medication and it builds up a resistance, therefore making the drug ineffective.[6]

Protozoans are single-celled organisms that can invade a human and cause disease. Three types of protozoans produce disease in humans: amoeba, flagellates, and sporozoans. *Entamoeba histolytica* is an amoeba that lives in the human intestinal tract without problem. However, if it invades the mucous membrane of the colon, it causes amoebic dysentery. *Giardia lamblia* is the flagellate that causes giardiasis, a type of diarrhea. This flagellate attaches itself to the surface of the small intestine and can become so prevalent that it interferes with nutrient absorption. Malaria is spread by mosquitoes carrying the sporozoa *Plasmodium*. *Plasmodium* multiplies in the liver and then invades the red blood cells, destroying them so extensively as to cause severe anemia.[7]

Healthcare-associated infections,[8] or **nosocomial infections**, are transmitted in hospitals, doctor's offices, and surgical clinics. Approximately two thirds of these infections are transmitted via central line pressure catheters, urinary catheters, and ventilators. A *Clostridium difficile* bacteria causing gastrointestinal infection can be transmitted to a patient by unclean hands.[9]

Community-acquired infections are those infections contracted through contact with people, animals, foods, water, etc., that are common in our environment. **Influenza** is a highly contagious community-

---

[4] www.cdc.gov/drugresistance/diseasesconnectedar.html

[5] www.news-medical.net/health/What-is-a-Virus.aspx

[6] www.news-medical.net/health/Human-Diseases-Caused-by-Viruses.aspx

[7] www.biologyreference.com/Po-Re/Protozoan-Diseases.html

acquired viral infection. Typically, symptoms of the flu occur 1–4 days after the virus enters the body. During this time, the host can transmit the infection to another person. [10]

Blood-borne pathogens are microorganisms that multiply in a human's bloodstream. These include hepatitis B, hepatitis C, and HIV. These types of infections are contracted through needle sticks, transfusions, and shared needles.

Transmission of Infection

Infections travel from one person to another in five ways:
1. Airborne/droplets;
2. Direct contact;
3. Indirect contact;
4. Vector method (animal); and
5. Fomite.

Airborne transmission occurs with a cough or sneeze. Some of the diseases transmitted in this fashion include influenza, mumps, pneumonia, tuberculosis, and meningitis.[11] The bacteria transmitted in this fashion are lightweight. Droplet transmission is a type of airborne transmission. The difference is the bacteria spread in this manner are too large to stay airborne for long.

Transmission via direct contact occurs when one person touches another person, as with handshaking, kissing, and sexual contact. A healthcare worker can transmit an infection from one patient to another via direct contact when safety precautions are not followed. Indirect contact occurs by touching an infected surface, such as a countertop.

Some diseases are transmitted from insects or animals, such as mosquitoes, ticks, and rodents. Examples are malaria and Lyme disease. The bubonic plague is transmitted by rats infected with *Yersinia pestis*.

Fomite bacterial transmission occurs when a bacterium on a nonliving object, such as bedding, towel, or a locker room, comes in contact with a person. The fungus *Trichophyton*, the source of athletes' foot, is transmitted from locker room floors.

---

[8] www.cdc.gov/hai/

[9] www.cdc.gov/HAI/infectionTypes.html

[10] www.cdc.gov/flu/about/disease/spread.htm

[11] http://www.biology.ed.ac.uk/archive/jdeacon/microbes/airborne.htm

Chain of Infection

Chain of infection refers to the steps necessary for bacteria, protozoa, fungi, and parasites to move from one person to another. There are six steps in the chain of infection: infectious agent, reservoir, portal of exit, mode of transmission, portal of entry, and susceptible host. All of these must be involved and in sequential (correct one-after-another) order to pass a disease from one person to another.

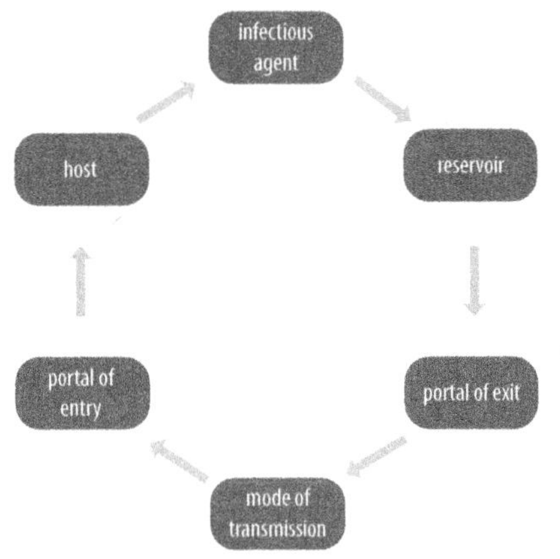

Infectious agent: The pathogen that causes the infection.

Here are some definitions you should know:

Reservoir: The area where the infectious agent can reproduce and multiply. This can be a person, animal, table top, door handle, etc.

Portal of exit: The manner in which the organism is released from the reservoir. This may be by coughing or sneezing or other method.

Mode of transmission: Cough, sneeze, handshake, touching an infected surface, using an infected towel, etc.

Port of entry: The point at which the pathogen enters another person. This could be through mucous membranes, open wounds, urinary catheters, or skin punctures from medical procedures, among others.

Susceptible host: A person or animal unable to resist the organism, allowing it in to multiply and cause a disease. This person has a compromised immune system, either from another disease or other debility.[12]

<hr>

[12] faculty.ccc.edu/tr-infectioncontrol/chain.htm

S.K.I.L.L. Check

What is the easiest portion of the chain of infection that can be broken?

Mode of transm [handwritten]

Notes:

Interrupting the chain of infection at any point stops the spread of disease. This is done by preventing the infectious agent from becoming airborne or a postoperative wound being properly bandaged to keep it clean. One of the easiest ways to break this chain is by hand washing.

Hand Washing

Hand washing is the easiest way to break the chain of infection. This applies to the general population and healthcare workers specifically. The Centers for Disease Control (CDC) recommends that healthcare workers wash their hands before any patient contact; after contact with blood, body fluids, or contaminated surfaces (even if gloves are worn); before invasive procedures; and after removing gloves (wearing gloves is not enough to prevent the transmission of pathogens in healthcare settings).[13] It is best to perform the hand washing in a patient's room so the patient can observe that you have done it.

To correctly wash your hands, the Mayo Clinic recommends the following procedure:
1. Wet your hands with running water.
2. Apply enough soap to cover the hands. Regular soap is as effective as antibacterial soap.
3. Lather well.
4. Rub the hands together, being sure to get soap to the backs of the hands, in between the fingers, and under the fingernails and wrists.
5. Rinse the soap from the hands.
6. Dry the hands with a single-use towel and use that towel to turn off the water.[14]

If soap and water are unavailable, using an alcohol-based hand cleaner is an acceptable alternative. This is called **hand rubbing**. An effective cleaner contains at least 60% alcohol. To clean your hands, the Mayo Clinic recommends the following:
1. Apply enough of the product to cover the hands.
2. Rub the hands together, covering all surfaces, until hands are dry.[15]

Hand washing is an important part of infection control, but there are also other ways to protect a healthcare worker from becoming infected.

---

[13] www.cdc.gov/handhygiene/Basics.html

[14] www.mayoclinic.com/health/hand-washing/HQ00407

[15] www.mayoclinic.com/health/hand-washing/HQ00407/NSECTIONGROUP=2

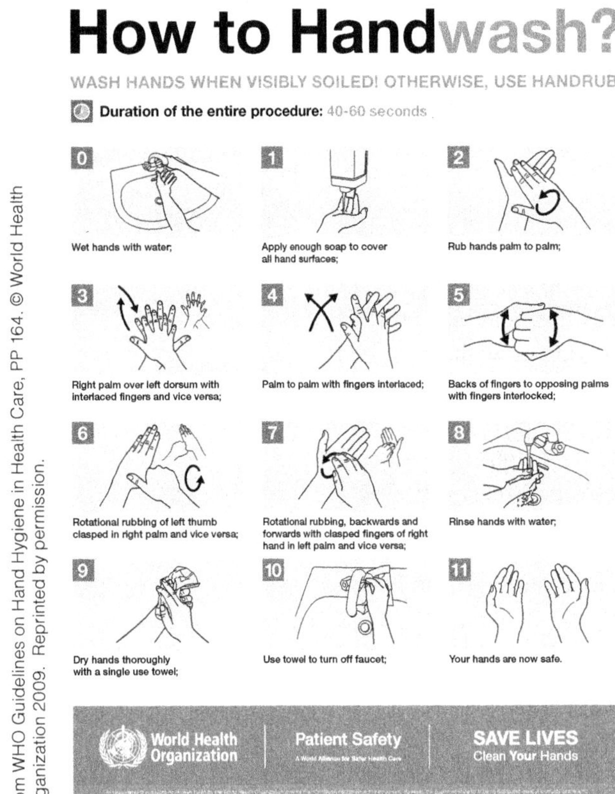

From WHO Guidelines on Hand Hygiene in Health Care, PP 164. © World Health Organization 2009. Reprinted by permission.

Protection from Infection

The Occupational Safety and Health Administration (OSHA) is the branch of government that's concerned with worker safety. In a healthcare setting, OSHA has developed guidelines to ensure prevention of contact with blood or other potentially infectious materials such as semen, vaginal secretions, amniotic fluid, saliva in dental procedures, etc. These guidelines are called "universal precautions" and apply to anyone working in any area where exposure to blood or other body fluids is likely.[16] Much of the universal precautions guidelines address what an employer must do to protect employees. This includes determining which jobs may potentially come into contact with blood-borne pathogens, providing the means to handle potential contaminations, providing personal protective equipment for all employees, managing the wastes produced in a hospital/nursing home environment, and providing hepatitis B vaccinations to all employees with risk of exposure.[17]

---

[16] www.osha.gov/SLTC/etools/hospital/hazards/ppe/ppe.html

[17] www.osha.gov/needlesticks/needlesticks-regtxtrev.html

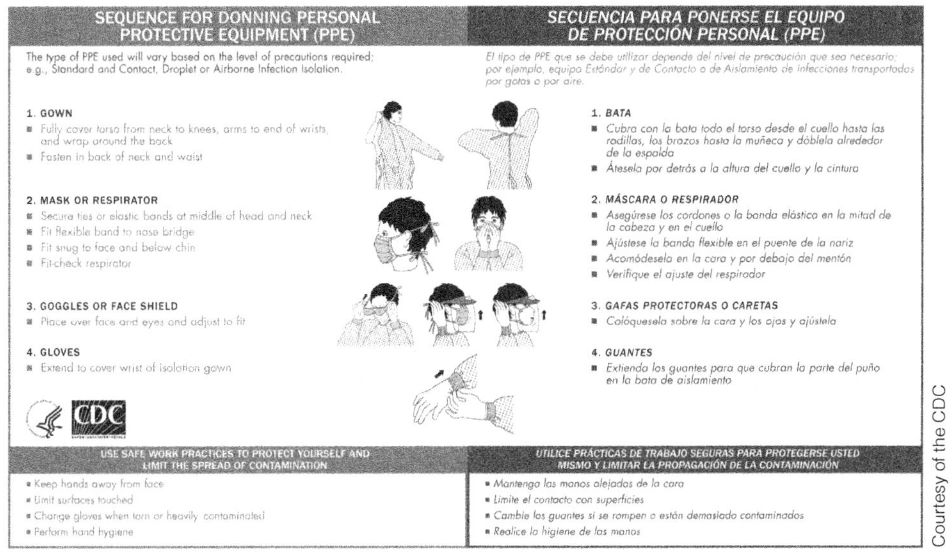

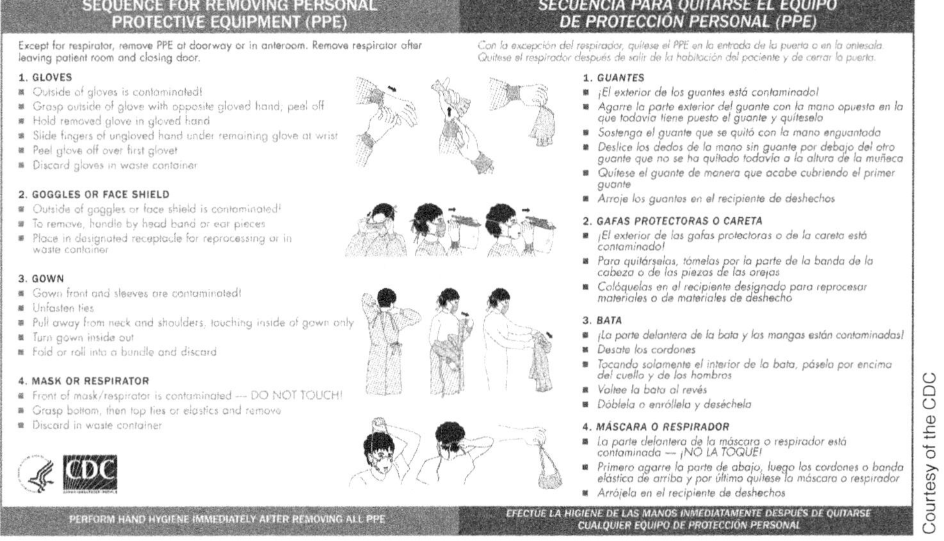

Personal protective equipment (PPE) must be provided by an employer. This includes such items such as gloves, face shields or masks, eye protection, and gowns and/or lab coats. Mouthpieces, resuscitation bags, and other ventilation devices must be made available.

To be termed "personal protective equipment" the device must not allow blood or other body fluids to touch an employee's skin, eyes, mouth, or clothing. Gloves are to be worn at any time it is conceivable that there may be contact with blood or other body fluids or contaminated surfaces. Face shields and masks must be worn any time there may be splashes, spray, or blood droplets, or other infectious material.

Each employer must have a set of procedures for using personal protective equipment, but the here are some general guidelines.

Eye and Face Protection: This includes a face mask covering the nose and mouth, and at other times, a mask to cover the entire face. Safety glasses may also need to be worn. These pieces of equipment are to protect the face and eyes from flying particles, liquid chemicals, and possible release of aerosol agents. The face protection also protects the employee from blood and body fluid contact.

Respirator: Some respirators protect the user by removing contaminants from the air (**particulate respirators**). Other respirators protect by providing clean air from an outside source. Respirators that provide clean air are **airline respirators**, using compressed air from a remote source and a self-contained breathing apparatus, which uses its own air supply. The workplace (hospital or clinic) will have a written process with worksite-specific procedures, including fitting of respirators, when to use the respirators, how to clean and disinfect the respirators, and how to use the respirators provided.[18] A properly fitting respirator allows the air pulled into the nose to enter only through the filter material of the respirator. Respirators of this type are used when working with patients with respiratory illnesses such as influenza or tuberculosis.

Surgical Masks: Surgical masks are physical barriers that protect the user from hazards such as large drops of blood or body fluids. Surgical masks cannot replace a respirator. A surgical mask protects the user from large contaminants, but cannot exclude the microscopic inhalants. Healthcare workers use the surgical mask to prevent contamination by patients and also to protect the patient from contamination by the healthcare worker. The surgical mask prevents organisms normally present in a healthcare worker's mucus and saliva from coming in contact with a patient's wounds. A mask prevents the user from placing contaminated fingers around the nose and mouth. Surgical masks can also be placed on a patient to prevent the patient from passing respiratory secretions to others.[19]

Hand Protection: The PPE for hand protection is gloves. The type of glove differs for different applications. For example, a laboratory technician may wear a single pair of disposable latex or nonlatex gloves when drawing blood from a patient. A surgeon may wear a double layer of nonlatex gloves during surgery. A housekeeper may wear vinyl gloves when emptying a hazardous waste disposal bin.

Laboratory Coats and Gowns: A lab coat or gown protects street clothes from biological or chemical spills, as well as provides some additional body protection. Scrubs are not considered PPE as they are worn like street clothes.[20]

Foot Protection: Generally, closed toed shoes must be worn in a healthcare setting. Sandals are not allowed due to potential exposure to hazardous fluids.

Other Areas of Protection

Sharps Containers: Blood-borne pathogens can be transmitted from a patient to a healthcare worker via needles and other sharp instruments. **Sharps** are needles, scalpels, broken glass, broken capillary tubes, and exposed ends of dental wires. All these may have come in contact with a pathogen, so all sharps must be safely disposed of. A sharps disposal container is available in a healthcare setting for used sharps. This must be closeable, upright, and stable during use, puncture resistant, leak proof at the sides and bottom, and

---

[18] OSHA Standards 29 CFR 1910, section 134, Respiratory Protection available at www.osha.gov/pls/oshaweb/owadisp.show_document?p_table=STANDARDS&p_id=12716

[19] OSHA Fact Sheet: Respiratory Infection Control: Respirators versus Surgical Masks retrieved from www.osha.gov/Publications/respirators-vs-surgicalmasks-factsheet.pdf

[20] Question #6 at www.osha.gov/pls/oshaweb/owadisp.show_document?p_table=INTERPRETATIONS&p_id=27008

properly labeled with the biohazard symbol and legend or color coded. The container must be clearly labeled that it contains sharp waste material.[21]

Laboratory Specimens: All specimens obtained from patients should be considered potentially infectious. As such, you must observe standard precautions for your protection. This includes:

- Wearing gloves when obtaining any specimen;
- Placing the specimen in an appropriate leak-proof container, taking care not to contaminate the outside of the container;
- Labeling the specimen appropriately; and
- Washing hands immediately after removing the gloves following a procedure.

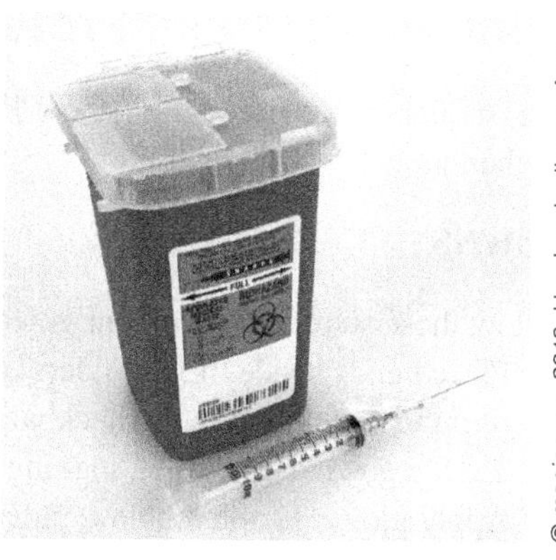

Laundry: Like lab specimens, all linens used by patients should be considered potentially infectious. Though the likelihood of spreading pathogens via used sheets is small, gowns and gloves must be worn when changing a patient bed. The sheets should be placed in a used linen hamper. Again, hands must be washed after handling linens.[22]

Medical Waste: The U.S. Environmental Protection Agency defines *medical waste* as "any solid waste that is generated in the diagnosis, treatment, or immunization of human beings or animals, in research pertaining thereto, or in the production or testing of biologicals, including but not limited to:

- Soiled or blood-soaked bandages
- Culture dishes and other glassware
- Discarded surgical gloves—after surgery
- Discarded surgical instruments—scalpels
- Needles—used to give shots or draw blood
- Cultures, stock, swabs used to inoculate cultures
- Removed body organs—tonsils, appendices, limbs, etc.
- Lancets"[23]

Currently, about 90 percent of medical waste is incinerated.[24] The EPA provides regulations for the disposal of medical wastes, as do individual states.

Personal Protective Equipment

Personal protective equipment (PPE) is designed to protect a healthcare worker from exposure to contaminants, such as blood, saliva, and other infectious materials. This generally includes gloves, gowns, masks, and eye/face protection. Which pieces of PPE you would wear depend on the type of exposure to infectious materials expected. Gloves are worn to protect the hands, gowns to protect skin and clothing, masks to protect mouth and nose, respirator to protect the respiratory tract from airborne infectious agents, goggles to protect the eyes, and face shields to protect the mouth, nose, eyes, and face.

---

[21] www.osha.gov/OshDoc/data_BloodborneFacts/bbfact02.pdf

[22] www.infectioncontroltoday.com/articles/2009/08/who-s-watching-the-laundry.aspx

[23] www.epa.gov/osw/nonhaz/industrial/medical/index.htm

[24] www.wastemed.com/treatment.htm

Donning Personal Protective Equipment

The sequence for putting on the PPE is (1) gown, (2) mask/respirator and eye and face protection, (3) then gloves.

GOWNS

Follow these steps to put on your gown:
1. Place hands inside the shoulders of the gown and move the gown to the body.
2. Slip the fingers inside the neckband to find the straps, then tie the gown at the back of the neck.
3. Tie the gown at the waist, making sure the gown covers the entire back of your uniform.
4. Apply gloves as noted below, pulling the cuffs of the gloves over the gown's sleeves to create a seal.

Follow these steps to remove the gloves and gown:
1. Remove gloves as noted below.
2. Untie the neck and back of the gown.
3. Slip the fingers of one hand under the sleeve of the other arm, pulling the sleeve down over the hand.
4. Using the hand covered by the sleeve, grasp the sleeve on the opposite side and pull the gown down to cover the hand.
5. With both hands inside the gown, remove the gown by grasping the shoulders and pulling it off.
6. Turn the gown inside out, keeping the contaminated surfaces on the inside. Roll it up and place in an appropriate receptacle.

If one gown is too small to cover you, use two gowns, one opening in the back and one opening in the front.

Mask: Place over nose, mouth, and chin. Fix flexible nose piece over the bridge of the nose. Secure it on your head using ties or elastic straps. Adjust to fit.

Particulate Respirator: This is put on like the mask, using a fit-tested respirator. Once the respirator is on, it should collapse on inhalation and it should not leak around face on exhalation.

Eye and Face Protection: Place the goggles over your eyes and secure it to your head with a headband or ear pieces. Put the face shield over your face and secure it with your headband. Adjust both to fit comfortably.

Nonsterile Gloves: These gloves should be available in all patient and examination rooms. Follow these steps to put them on:
1. Wash your hands.
2. Remove a pair of the appropriately sized gloves from the container. Touch only the gloves to be used. As these are nonsterile gloves, there is no standard procedure for putting them on.

Sterile Gloves

Follow these steps to put on sterile gloves
1. Wash your hands following the standard procedure.
2. Inspect the glove packaging to ensure there are no tears or stains. If found, do not use the gloves.
3. Place the gloves on a clean, dry, flat surface at about waist height.
    a. The gloves should be facing away from the body, with the palms and thumbs up.
    b. If not in this position, rotate the package so the gloves are in the proper position, taking care to not touch the inner lining of the packaging and don't reach over the gloves.

4. Without touching the sterile inner lining, open the glove package by pulling the tabs.
5. Pick up the first glove at the top edge of the folded down cuff. Do not drag the glove or touch the outside of the glove.
6. Hold the glove above the waist and slip fingers in, pulling it on by holding onto the inside cuff.
7. Using the gloved hand, slip the fingers inside the cuff of the other glove, then slip your fingers into the glove.
8. Adjust the gloves for a proper fit, being careful to not touch your skin with the gloved hands.
9. Slide fingers under the cuff and push cuff back to cover the wrists.
10. Check for any flaws or imperfections in the gloves. If found, remove the gloves and start over.

Removing Personal Protective Equipment

Any area of the PPE that may have been in contact with possibly infectious materials is considered the "contaminated side." Areas that are considered "clean" would be inside, outside back, ties on head and back—any area likely not to have been in contact with infectious areas. The sequence for removing PPE is (1) gloves, (2) face/eye protection, (3) gown, and (4) mask/respirator. PPE should be removed at the door of the patient's room, removing the mask/respirator outside of the patient room.

Gloves: Grasp outside edge of glove near the wrist, peel the glove off the hand, turning it inside out, holding the first glove in the opposite gloved hand. Slide the ungloved finger under the wrist edge of the remaining glove; peel the glove off the hand, keeping the first glove in the palm, creating a bag for both gloves. Discard appropriately.

Eye and Face Protection: Grasp the ear or head pieces with your ungloved hands, lifting the protective gear away from the face. Discard appropriately.

Gown: Unfasten the ties. Pull the gown off shoulders and arms, folding the contaminated side toward the inside, creating a bundle or roll. Discard appropriately.

Mask: Untie the bottom tie, then the top tie. Remove it from your face. Discard appropriately.

Particulate Respirator: Lift bottom elastic over top of your head. Then lift the top elastic. Discard appropriately.

Immediately wash your hands after removing the personal protective equipment.

When to Use PPE

Gloves: Use gloves when you anticipate touching blood, body fluids, secretions, excretions, or contaminated items. Also wear gloves when touching mucus membranes and nonintact skin.

Gowns: Wear gowns during procedures and patient care activities when you anticipate contact of clothing or exposed skin with blood or body fluids, secretions, or excretions.

Mask and Goggles or a Face Shield: Wear a mask and goggles or wear a face shield during patient care activities likely to generate splashes or sprays of blood, body fluids, secretions, or excretions.[25]

---

[25] The information above about PPE taken from a PowerPoint presentation titled "Guidance for the Selection and Use of Personal Protective Equipment (PPE) in Healthcare Settings" from the CDC at www.cdc.gov/HAI/ppt/ppe/PPEslides6-29-04.ppt.

Asepsis

Asepsis refers to the lack of bacteria, viruses, and other microorganisms. There are two categories of asepsis: surgical and general. **Surgical asepsis** refers to decontamination of equipment and personnel prior to, during, and following an invasive surgical procedure. Surgical asepsis includes setting up a sterile field in the operating room, which means the equipment must be sterilized and personnel must practice sterile technique. **General asepsis** refers to caring for patients outside of the operating room.

In the 1960s Earle Spaulding devised an approach to disinfection and sterilization of patient care items. Equipment that must be aseptic can be categorized in three degrees: critical, semicritical, and noncritical.[26] Critical items are those objects that enter sterile tissue or the vascular system such as surgical instruments, urinary and cardiac catheters, implants, and ultrasound probes used in sterile body cavities. Semicritical items are objects that touch mucuous membranes or nonintact skin. This includes respiratory therapy and anesthesia equipment, some endoscopes, cystoscopes, etc. Noncritical equipment refers to objects that come into contact with intact skin but not mucous membranes. Noncritical items are further divided into patient-care items and noncritical environmental surfaces. Items such as blood pressure cuffs, bedpans, crutches, and computers in the noncritical patient-care category. Noncritical environmental surfaces include bed rails, bedside tables, patient furniture, floors, and some food utensils.

The classification of equipment dictates what type of sterilization or disinfecting must be done. The methods used include heat sterilization, ethylene oxide or hydrogen peroxide gas, hydrogen peroxide, isopropyl alcohol, and germicidal detergent solutions.[27]

When equipment has been sterilized, it is packaged with an indicator that changes when the sterilization boundary has been broken. This may be a strip within the packaging that changes color when sterilization is complete or a glass vial containing pellets that melt when sterilization has occurred. When the equipment is no longer sterilized, it must not be used and needs to be sent back for resterilization.

Sterile Technique

Certain steps must be followed to ensure that sterilized equipment remains sterile. These guidelines state that:
- You must always wear gloves.
- You may never reach across the sterile field.
- Inner packaging is considered sterile; the outside is not.

---

[26] www.cdc.gov/hicpac/pdf/guidelines/Disinfection_Nov_2008.pdf

[27] Rutala & Weber, 2008, Guidelines for Disinfection and Sterilization in Healthcare Facilities, Healthcare Infection Control Practices Advisory Committee, CDC.

- The edges of trays are not sterile.
- You must keep your hands above the table.
- The sterile field extends 1½ inches beyond the equipment.
- You may touch the equipment in the package only once with gloved hands.

Instruments to be used in a procedure must be in a sterile package. When opening a sterile pack, follow these steps.

1. Wash your hands and put on sterile gloves.
2. Establish a sterile field by opening a sterile drape from a corner, allowing it to hang free, and placing it on a flat surface without touching the inside of the drape.
3. Place the sterile pack on a clean, flat surface so the top flap will open in an upward fashion.
4. Open the top flap, the left flap, the right flap, and bottom flap. A sterile field has now been created. Do not cross over this area.
5. Open the top flap of the inner layer, then the left, right, and bottom flap.
6. Check the sterilization indicator inside the pack. If it indicates the pack is not sterile, do not use it. Open another sterile pack.
7. Cover the instrument(s) with a sterile sheet.[28]
8. If instrument hands are not facing the user, rotate the entire pack on the table, using the corners of the outer packaging to move the supplies.

If the material to be used comes in a commercially prepared sterile pack, peel the package open and drop the instruments onto a sterile field. The inside of the packaging is considered sterile and can be used to create a sterile field. However, the outside of the packaging is not sterile and should not touch a sterile field.[29]

Placing fluids on a sterile field may need to be done during a procedure. Follow these steps to place the fluids on a sterile field:

1. Wash your hands.
2. Put on sterile gloves.
3. Keep the fluid container out of the sterile field.
4. Hold the bottle in your dominant hand with the label facing the palm of your hand.
5. Remove the bottle cap, making sure to not touch the inner rim of the bottle with the outside of the cap.
6. Pour a small amount of liquid into an emesis basin to clean off the lip of the bottle.
7. Pick up the sterile container in which to pour the fluid and step back from the sterile field.
8. Hold the bottle about 6 inches above the container into which the fluid is to be poured. Pour the liquid in a slow, steady stream to prevent splashing. Do not allow the lip of the bottle to touch the container and do not pass the bottle over the sterile field.
9. Replace the container on the sterile field.
10. Recap the bottle.[30]

With any procedure there is some hazardous waste. This might be fluids, sharps, linens, or instruments. Place sharps into a sharps container. Remove linens from the field, enclosing the contaminated area within the bundle and then place the bundle into a contaminated waste container. Instruments should be returned to the hospital central supply area for resterilization and repackaging. Single-use instruments should be

---

[28] www.russpowell.com/wksamples/USCG_HS_HowToOpenSterilePack.pdf

[29] www.austincc.edu/adnlev1/rnsg1413skillslab/sterile_technique/notes_surg_asepsis.htm

[30] nursing411.org/Courses/MD0540_Sterile_Procedures/3-06_Sterile_Procedures.html

disposed of according to manufacturer recommendations. All this is done to ensure that potential contaminants have been removed from patient care areas.

Working in a healthcare setting can be hazardous to one's health, but there are ways to minimize the risk of exposure to blood-borne and airborne pathogens. Knowing what causes infections, how pathogens can be transmitted, and how to prevent the transmission of pathogens protects both you and the patient.

Exercises

Key Information Memory (K.I.M.)

Use this graphic organizer to consolidate information and provide an easier way to relate the vocabulary with a definition by using a visual aid in a more familiar context to help identify the subject, definition, and concept. By placing the vocabulary word in one column, then writing the definition in the next, the user selects a memory cue to draw in the third column.

Chapter 3 *Questions*

1. What is *normal* flora?

2. What is a *protozoa*? Name the three types of protozoa that cause diseases in humans.

3. What is the difference between a *nosocomial infection* and a *community-acquired infection*?

4. What is a *fomite transmission of infection*?

5. Name the six steps of the infectious process. What happens if one of these steps is missing?

6. What is the easiest way to break the chain of infection? Describe how to do this.

7. What are *universal precautions*? Who developed these?

8. Personal protective equipment is provided by an employer. What is personal protective equipment?

9. What is a *sharps container*? What color is this piece of equipment?

10. What is the proper sequence for putting on personal protective equipment?

Patient Mobility

Hospitalized patients spend the majority of their time in bed. It is important to be aware of the position the patient is in while lying in bed and possible complications associated with the position. The goal of any hospitalization is patient discharge. Mobilizing the patient is important in achieving this goal. However, patients cannot simply be made to stand up and be told to walk. The physical condition of the patient or the type of procedure performed on the patient determine how he or she should be mobilized. This involves transferring the patient from one position to another, which needs to be done with the safety of the patient foremost. Studies have shown that patient mobility speeds up recovery time and shortens hospital stays.[1,2]

Patient Positioning

The position a patient lies in is important to his or her overall condition and affects his or her hospital discharge. There are different ways to have a patient lie down or sit some—related to the procedure the patient may have undergone and some the patient will assume on his or her own. The common positions are supine, prone, lateral, Sims, Fowlers, Trendelenburg, orthopneic, litihotomy, and sitting.

The **supine** position means the patient is lying on his back. The opposite of supine is **prone**, meaning the patient is lying face down. The **lateral** position means the patient is lying on her side, either the right or left. These are positions the patient may assume on his own.

A patient is in the **Sims** position is lying on the left side and chest with the right knee and thigh drawn up and the left arm along the back. This position is commonly used to perform rectal examinations.[3]

S.K.I.L.L. Check

Patient positioning is primarily for what purpose?

promote mobility & speed recovery time

Notes:

---

[1] archinte.jamanetwork.com/article.aspx?articleid=1106282

[2] onlinelibrary.wiley.com/doi/10.1111/j.1532-5415.2010.03276.x/abstract

[3] armymedical.tpub.com/MD0906/MD09060013.htm

See www.healthmango.com/wp-content/uploads/2010/02/sims-position.jpg to see a picture of Sims position

In the **Fowler's** position, the head of the bed is elevated 30–90 degrees and the knees are also elevated. This position is commonly used to promote easy breathing and drainage.[4]

See medical-dictionary.thefreedictionary.com/position for a picture of Fowler's position

In the **Trendelenberg** position, the patient is supine on a surface inclined 45 degrees, with the head at the lower end and legs flexed over the upper end. This position is used when inserting or removing central venous catheters, for pelvic and gynecologic surgery or abdominal hernia reduction, and during delivery when a cord prolapse occurs.[5]

See http://upload.wikimedia.org/wikipedia/commons/3/36/Trendelenburg_position.gif to see a picture of Trendelenburg position.

When a patient has shortness of breath exacerbated (made worse) by lying down, she is put in an **orthopneic** position. In this position, the patient is an upright or semivertical position using pillows to support the head and chest, or the patient sits upright in a chair.

See jpkc.fimmu.com/hl/Course/Content/n1045/200506212032/woweitu/duanzuowei3.JPG to see a picture of a patient in the orthopneic position

The **Lithotomy** position occurs when the patient is placed supine on a surface with the legs well separated, hips and knees each bent to 90 degrees and thighs bent outward from the hips. Stirrups may be used to support the feet and legs.

Picture from upload.wikimedia.org/wikipedia/commons/thumb/d/d6/Lithotomy_position.jpg/220px-Lithotomy_position.jpg

Sitting position occurs when a patient is placed in a chair or the head of the bed is placed at a 90 degree angle.

Each position comes with different pressure point areas. The supine, prone, lateral, and sitting positions cause the most concern because patients will remain in these positions for long periods. A patient in a certain position for an extended time may develop decubitus ulcers (bedsores). To prevent the bedsores, pressure points need to be padded. A **pressure point** is a place where the patient's bones are most visible and they press against other body parts, mattress, or chair.

When in the supine position, pressure points include the back of the head, elbows, scapula (shoulder blades), pelvic area, and heels. The prone position pressure points are the ear, cheek, acromion (highest point of the shoulder), breasts, iliac crest (upper bony margin of the pelvis), male genitalia, patella (kneecap), and toes. In the lateral position, pressure points are the elbows, acromion, the iliac crest, greater trochanter (top of the femur, on the side), medial and lateral condyles (projections of the femur at the inside and outside of the knee), and medial and lateral malleoli (projections of the tibia at the inside and outside of the ankle).[6] Pressure points in the sitting position include the scapula, ischial tuberosities (bones of the sacrum that are felt when sitting), back of the knees, and calcanei (heels). These points need to be padded to prevent bedsores.

---

[4] armymedical.tpub.com/MD0906/MD09060012.htm

[5] www.slideshare.net/akhlak21/trendelenburg-position

[6] www.pfiedler.com/1079/1079.pdf

Dedubitus ulcers (bedsores) develop when there is pressure over a bony surface, causing the skin to wear away. The first stage of a bedsore is skin reddening, which does not go away when the pressure is removed. A second-degree bedsore is loss of the top layers of skin. Third-degree bedsores occur with full thickness skin loss. Fourth-degree bedsores are full thickness skin loss with destruction of underlying muscle, bone, and/or supporting structures. You can prevent bedsores by padding the pressure points; however, patient movement is the best prevention.

Other complications of patient immobility include contractures and muscle atrophy. Contractures, or shortening of muscles so they cannot be easily moved, occur when the muscles aren't being used and the nonbony tissues such as muscles, tendons, ligaments, and skin become inelastic. **Muscle atrophy** occurs when muscles aren't used and decrease in size. Muscle and joint movement helps to prevent these complications.

Transferring Patients

Hospitalized patients must be moved from one location to another for procedures and keep them mobile. Most often patients are transferred from a bed to a wheelchair, walker, or gurney. There are several safe ways to transfer patients.

When transferring a patient, you need to consider several items before moving. Is the patient independently mobile (does the patient move on his or her own)? Has the patient had a joint replacement? Does the patient have a history of falls? Does the patient have a catheter? Has the patient had a fracture? Does the patient have any respiratory or cardiac impairment? Also, how much does the patient weight? If a patient weighs more than 25% of your body weight, a second person is needed for the transfer. All these questions and more need to be considered.[7]

Before starting a transfer, make sure there is plenty of room for the equipment needed. Ask the patient if he or she is independently mobile. If not, ask her what side of the body is stronger. It is best to transfer the patient to the strongest side of her body.

Equipment used in transfers may include a gait (transfer) belt and a sliding (transfer) board.

A **gait (transfer) belt** is a device used to move a patient from one place to another and avoid injury to both caregiver and patient in the process. Gait belts come in different sizes and padding. The most common belt has metal claps and is made of canvas. A gait belt is placed around the patient's waist and used to balance the patient while standing and turning or walking. It is not used to lift a patient.

---

[7] cas.umkc.edu/casww/transfrg.htm[4] medical-dictionary.thefreedictionary.com/fever

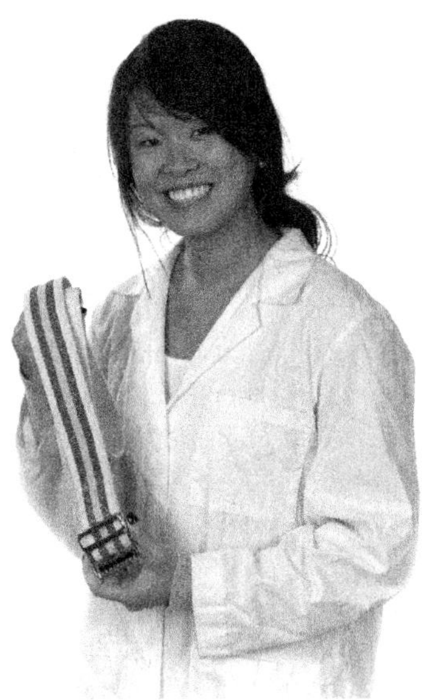

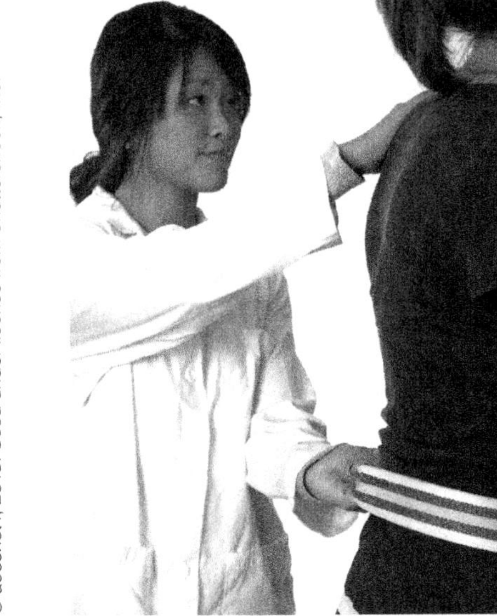

A **sliding (transfer) board** is made of flexible plastic and may have hand holes around the sides. This is used to help the patient move from bed to a wheelchair, a wheelchair to a toilet, or a wheelchair to a car.

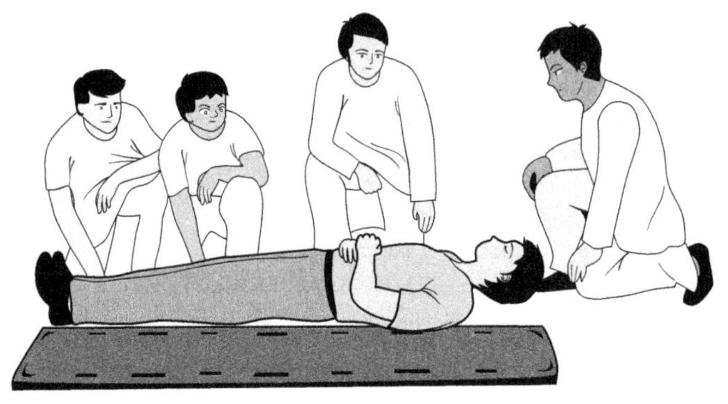

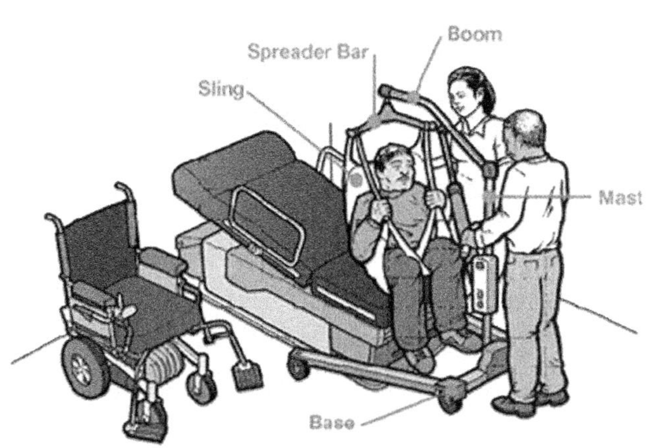

Picture from http://www.fda.gov/MedicalDevices/ProductsandMedicalProcedures/GeneralHospital DevicesandSupplies/ucm308622.htm

For heavy patients, a patient lift may be used. These devices enable transfer of a patient using a sling. They can be powered manually or with a power source such as a battery. The sling is slid under the patient and a boom raises the sling to provide clearance so the patient can be moved from the bed to a chair or toilet.

To transfer a patient from the bed to a wheelchair, follow these steps:[8]
1. Tell the patient why he is to be moved and how it will be done. If the patient can move by himself, stand by his side to provide assistance as necessary.
2. Before he moves to the wheelchair, make sure the brake is on and the footrests are removed or placed in an upright position. If possible, remove the armrest from the side closest to the bed.
3. Stabilize the bed so it won't move and lower it until it's level with the wheelchair seat. Be aware of any tubes or catheters the patient may have that could hinder the transfer.
4. Place the wheelchair at a slight angle beside the bed, with the seat close to the bed.
5. Put nonskid booties on the patient's feet.
6. Move the patient to the edge of the bed and move his legs over the side, with his knees near the edge of the bed.
7. Have the patient put his hands in his lap.
8. Grasp the patient around the chest, under the armpits.
9. Assist the patient to a sitting position and hold on until he can sit without support.
10. For assistance in moving the patient, you can put a transfer belt around his waist.

---

[8] www.nlm.nih.gov/medlineplus/ency/patientinstructions/000428.htm

11. Gradually slide the patient forward until his feet are on the floor. Place your feet on either side of the patient's feet, far enough apart to give yourself a good base of support.
12. Have the patient lean forward, placing his arms around your shoulders. Have him reach for the far arm of the wheelchair.
13. Place your arms around the patient's wait, gripping the transfer belt toward the back. Be sure to keep your back straight as you bend your hips and knees.
14. Keeping the patient's knees stabilized, count to 3 and on 3 pull forward on the belt to lift him.
15. When the patient is high enough to clear the armrest or chair surface, turn, taking small steps, while keeping the patient's knees blocked with your knees.
16. When you have the patient turned, bend your hips to lower the patient into the chair.
17. Replace footrest and armrests and remove the transfer belt.
18. Fasten the seatbelt on the wheelchair.

Follow these steps to transfer a patient from a wheelchair to the bed:
1. Set the brake on the wheelchair so it won't move.
2. Stabilize the bed so it won't move and lower it to the floor.
3. Put a transfer belt around the patient's waist.
4. Stand in front of the patient.
5. With a straight back, bend from the hips and knees and grasp the patient around the waist, holding onto the transfer belt.
6. Stand erect pulling the patient up, keeping her knees between your knees.
7. Pause to make sure the patient is stable.
8. Taking small steps, pivot the patient so her back is square with the bed.
9. Slowly lower the patient to the bed, bending your knees and hips.
10. Swing the patient's legs onto the bed and help her return to the recumbent position.

A transfer (slide) board can make the transfer from a bed to a wheelchair easier by providing some support to the patient while moving. To transfer a patient from bed to wheelchair using a slide board, follow these steps:[9]
1. Tell the patient why he is to be moved and how it will be done. If the patient can move on his own, stand by his side to provide assistance as necessary.
2. Before he moves to the wheelchair, make sure the brake is on and the footrests are removed or placed in an upright position. If possible, remove the armrest from the side closest to the bed.
3. Stabilize the bed so it won't move and lower it until it's level with the wheelchair seat. Be aware of any tubes or catheters the patient may have that could hinder the transfer.
4. Place the wheelchair at a slight angle beside the bed, with the seat close to the bed.
5. Place the slide board so it bridges the gap between the bed and wheelchair. One third of the board needs to be on the wheelchair seat, one third across the gap, with the remaining third resting firmly on the bed. You could place a sheet on the board to help the patient slide and to protect his skin.
6. Help the patient into a sitting position and hold on to him until he can sit without support.
7. Put a transfer belt around the patient's waist.
8. Position the board under the patient's hip closest to the wheelchair, holding on to the transfer belt.

---

[9] http://www.ehow.com/how_6108732_use-sliding-transfer-board.html#ixzz2GwbmMuCa

9. Instruct the patient reach for the far arm of the wheelchair for support and push on the bed with the other hand while helping the patient move across the board.

10. When the patient is in the wheelchair, remove the board from under the patient's hip.

11. Replace the wheelchair armrest and replace or lower the footrests.[10]

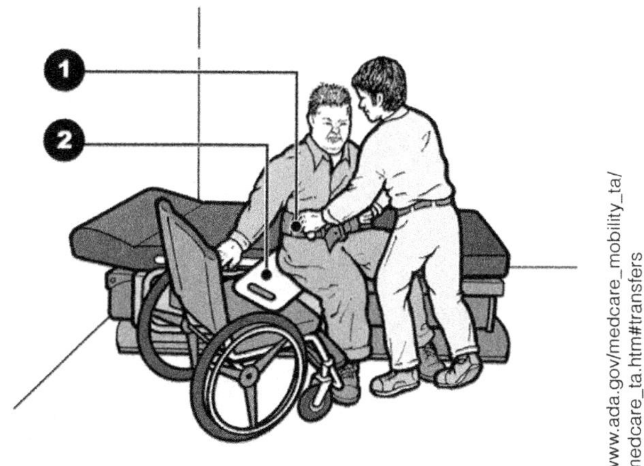

(1) Gait or transfer belt; (2) Slide or transfer board. Picture from www.ada.gov/medcare_mobility_ta/medcare_ta.htm#transfers

Safety Guidelines

Patient safety must be foremost in the minds of healthcare workers. This includes making sure the patient is safe in bed, safe when ambulating, and safe when in the bathroom.

Hospital beds are equipped with side rails that keep a patient from rolling out of bed. Side rails are not to be used as restraints. If a patient is capable of harming him- or herself, another form of restraint should be used. Beds are provided with a call button that the patient can use to summon nursing personnel for assistance. The call button is also used to move the bed up and down, capable of moving the head and foot ends independently.

---

[10] Information regarding transfers obtained from www.nlm.nih.gov/medlineplus/ency/patientinstructions/000428.htm; www.mtpinnacle.com/pdfs/Guide-to-Safe-Patient-Handling.pdf; www.ehow.com/how_2311857_transfer-weak-patient-from-bed.html; www.drugs.com/cg/wheel-chair-transfers.html

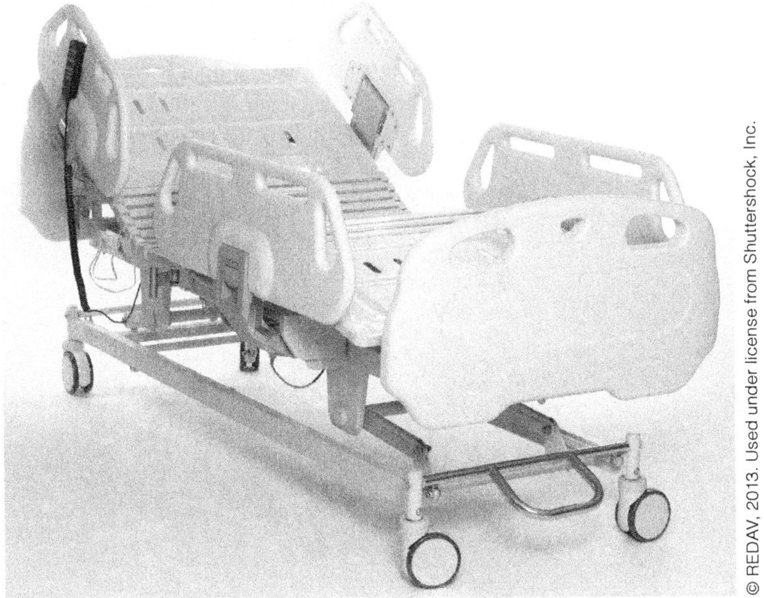

© REDAV, 2013. Used under license from Shuttershock, Inc.

Hospital beds can trap patients. Entrapment is uncommon but the possibility needs to be addressed. The FDA (U.S. Food and Drug Administration) has identified seven areas of entrapment:

1. within the rail;
2. under the rail, between the rail supports, or next to a single rail support;
3. between the rail and the mattress;
4. between the rail, at the ends of the rail;
5. between split bed rails;
6. between the end of the rail and the side edge of the head or foot board; and
7. between the head- or footboard and the mattress end.[11]

The patient should be positioned in the bed so there is little chance of moving into a position where entrapment in the above areas is possible. If it's possible for the patient to move into a position where there would be entrapment, restraints may be needed.

Bathrooms are another place where patient safety is a concern. Because of the risk of falls, hospitals must follow specific guidelines when the bathrooms are constructed. These guidelines are outlined in the description of Water Closets on the ADA Accessibility Guidelines for Buildings and Facilities.[12] Hospital bathrooms must be large enough for someone to assist a patient when using the toilet and shower. The flooring must be slip resistant. Needless to say, patients accessing bathrooms increase the incidence of falls so caregivers must be aware of patient location and alert to patient toileting needs.

---

[11] www.fda.gov/downloads/ForConsumers/ConsumerUpdates/UCM164395.pdf

[12] www.access-board.gov/adaag/html/adaag.htm#4.16

Restraints

At times, a patient may appear to be in a state that requires the use of restraints. Patient restraints are typically used to prevent patient falls and wandering, protect equipment, and control agitation. Restraints are also used to prevent risk of injury or harm to others. Physical restraints include ankle ties, roll belts, and wrist ties. Chemical restraints include the administration of sedative and anti-anxiety medications to calm a patient and allow a medical treatment to be given. Environmental restraints limit the area in which a patient may move, such as being confined to a room to prevent wandering. Monitoring devices such as a bed alarm can also be used to monitor the patient's movement. Restraints are used only after assessing the patient and trying other, less restrictive types of behavior control.[13,14]

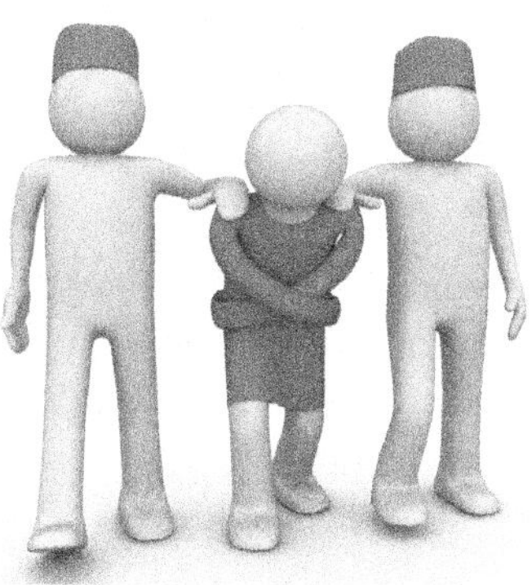

Restraints can be made of hard or soft materials. Soft mitts prevent a patient from being able to grasp things, but still able to move his or her arms. Lap belts are used to decrease the risk of a fall by stopping a patient from getting up and out of a chair. A roll belt prevents a patient from getting out of bed. Soft wrist restraints prevent a patient from pulling at an IV or other tube or removing a dressing.

Soft foam wrist or ankle restraints are cloth straps closed with Velcro or a thread-through buckle. These are placed on the patient and secured to the bed frame, leaving enough room so when the bed is raised, the restraint does not impair circulation.

Belt restraints are wrapped around a patient and closed at the patient's back. These are attached to the bed or chair frame.

S.K.I.L.L. Check

Restraints are for what two purposes?

[handwritten: Prevent injury/harm to self or others]

Notes:

---

[13] www.drugs.com/cg/the-medical-use-of-restraints.html

[14] www.hamiltonhealthsciences.ca/documents/Patient%20Education/PatientRestraint-trh.pdf

Vest restraints are canvas or mesh jackets that are placed around the patient and secured to the bed or chair frame. The opening of this type of restraint is in the front and looks like a vest worn with a suit. The straps cross at the bottom of the vest and attach to the side of the bed or wheelchair.

Mitts are wrapped around a patient's hands and secured above the wrist. This prevents a patient from pulling at or removing catheters but allows arm movement.[15]

Conclusion

Keeping patients mobile while in the hospital decreases recovery time, but mobility must be tempered with safety measures. Restraints help keep a patient safe, gait belts help you transfer a patient from bed to chair, and positioning a patient while in bed adds to their safe recovery. Safety must always be foremost in the minds of healthcare workers.

SKILL Check Activity

Key Information Memory (K.I.M.)

Use this graphic organizer to consolidate information and provide an easier way to relate the vocabulary with a definition by using a visual aid in a more familiar context in which to help identify the subject, definition, and concept. By placing the vocabulary word in one column, then writing the definition in the next, the user selects a memory cue to draw in the third column.

---

[15] Ellis & Nowlis. *Modules for basic nursing skills: Vol. 1*, (pp. 421–424). Atlanta Book Co.

Chapter 4 *Questions*

1. Describe the Fowler's position. *Head of bed is elevated 30-90° - knees also elevated*

2. Why would a patient be put into an orthopneic position? *When a pt has SOB exacerbated by lying down*

3. Name three reasons why a patient may be put into restraints. *Prevent falls, protect equip, control agitation*

4. Describe moving a patient from a wheelchair to bed. *Set brake on W.C, stabilize, lower bed, Trfr belt around pt waist, stand in front pt, bend from hips - grasp pt around waist Pqsu*

5. What would be the best way to move a patient who weighs more than 300 pounds? *Pt lift*

6. Why would a patient be put into the Sims position? *For rectal exam*

7. What is a *decubitus ulcer*? What causes this condition? How can it be treated? *Bedore caused by pressure points press against pt, other body matterss prevention by padding press. pts - pt movement*

8. Why is a gait belt used? *To help balance pt while standing & turning or walking.*

Chapter 5

Special Care: Physiologic Needs, Support Equipment, Hospital Safety

Patients need assistance with physiological needs while in a hospital. During a hospital stay, patients may need help with bowel movements, urination, oronasal secretion removal, cardiac and/or respiratory collapse, oxygen therapy, and drainage tubes/catheters. Each function has specific equipment.

Bedpans/Urinals

Bedpans are containers used by patients when they have a bowel movement or urinate while confined to bed. Both men and women use the bedpan for a bowel movement, and a woman uses the bedpan to urinate. A man generally uses a hand-held urinal when urinating. There are urinals designed for women to use also.

Helping a Patient Use a Bedpan

Have the following items within easy reach: a basin with warm water, gloves, toilet paper, washcloths and towels.
1. Run warm water over the bedpan to remove the chill. If using a metal bedpan, make sure the metal is not so hot that it would burn the patient.
2. Sprinkle baby powder on the edge of the bedpan to make it easier for the patient to slide onto it.
3. Wash hands and put on the gloves.
4. Slide a waterproof pad under the patient.

5. Support the patient's lower back while sliding the edge of the bedpan under his buttocks.
6. Raise the head of the bed to enable the patient to reach a sitting position. This aids the patient in moving the bowels or urinating.
7. Give the patient privacy if possible. If the patient is weak, do not leave him alone.
8. When the patient is done, lower the head of the bed and ask the patient to raise his buttocks while you remove the pan. Cover the pan with a towel and place it on a chair next to the bed.
9. Gently roll the patient onto his side and clean his buttocks with toilet paper.
10. Use a wet washcloth to clean the area, using soap and water if necessary. (If the patient is female, clean from front to back.)
11. Dry between the patient's legs.

Helping a Patient Use a Urinal

1. Ask the patient to place the urinal between her legs. If the patient is unable to so, spread her legs and put the urinal in place. (If the patient is male, ask him to put his penis in the opening at the top of the urinal. If unable to do so, assist him in positioning his penis.)
2. Position the urinal properly and hold it gently while the patient urinates.
3. When finished, carefully remove the urinal, cover it with a towel and place it on a chair next to the bed.
4. Assist the patient in cleaning between the legs with a damp washcloth. (If the patient is female, clean from front to back.)
5. Dry the area between the legs.

After Using the Bedpan or Urinal

1. Give the patient a damp washcloth to clean her hands.
2. Take the bedpan/urinal to the bathroom and empty it into the toilet.
3. Clean the bedpan/urinal with soap and water using a toilet brush. Then disinfect the bedpan/urinal.[1]

Emesis Basin

An **emesis basin** is a small, kidney-shaped receptacle (usually plastic) used to catch vomitus. However, these are often inadequate to the task so an **emesis bag** is used instead. This is a long plastic bag with a rigid collar and a one-way valve at the mouth of the bag. Once used, the bag can be twisted closed and disposed of.

Oral Suctioning

Oral suctioning is done when a patient is unable to clear secretions from the mouth and throat. This is a procedure that can be traumatic for the patient, so care must be taken to ensure it is done properly.

---

[1] www.drugs.com/cg/helping-someone-use-a-bedpan-or-a-urinal.html

Performing Oral Sunctioning

Have the following equipment on hand: suction unit, sterile suction catheters, wide-bore rigid suctioning tubes (if ordered for the patient), gloves, and protective eye wear, and oxygen (if ordered). Explain the procedure to the patient and gain her consent.

1. Wash hands and put on the gloves, apron, and protective eye wear.
2. Turn on the suction apparatus and set the pressure to an appropriate level.
3. Attach the suction catheter or suction tube to the suction apparatus.
4. Ask the patient open her mouth so the secretions are visible.
5. Insert the suction catheter or tube into the patient's mouth along one cheek.
6. Turn the suction apparatus inward and gently remove secretions from one side of the mouth. Repeat on the other side of the mouth.
7. Evaluate the color, amount, and consistency of the secretions and document the information on the patient's chart.
8. Clean the suction catheter/tube by sucking sterile water through the tube until the tube is clear.
9. Dispose of your gloves and remove your apron and protective eye wear.
10. Make sure the patient is comfortable.[2]
11. Administer oxygen before and after the procedure if ordered.

Nasal Suctioning

This procedure is performed on patients who may have a decreased level of consciousness, muscle weakness, or an inability to clear secretions and maintain a patent or open airway. This is an unpleasant procedure for the patient and should only be performed as a last resort.

Gather the following equipment: suction unit, sterile suction catheters, sterile lubricant, bag-valve mask, basin of warm water, gloves, protective eye wear, and oxygen (if ordered).

1. Explain procedure to the patient and gain consent.
2. Wash your hands and put on the gloves, gown, and protective eye wear.
3. Turn on the suction apparatus and set the pressure to an appropriate level.
4. Keeping the catheter inside its sterile bag, attach the correctly sized catheter to the suction apparatus.
5. Hold the exposed catheter in your dominant hand and remove the packaging, making sure the catheter does not touch anything.
6. Dip the tip of the catheter into the sterile gel and insert the tip into the patient's nostril without turning on the suction pressure.
7. Advance the catheter to the back of the nose until you feel resistance.
8. Rotate the catheter between your thumb and index finger until you overcome the resistance..
9. Ask the patient to take a deep breath while you advance the catheter. This helps the catheter enter the trachea.
10. Begin withdrawing the catheter while applying suction pressure, removing the catheter from the nostril. This should take about 10–15 seconds.
11. Release the suction and wrap your dominant hand around the catheter.

---

[2] Randle, Coffey & Bradbury (eds.). (2009). *Oxford handbook of clinical skills in adult nursing* (310). Oxford: Oxford University Press.

12. Invert your glove around the catheter and appropriately dispose of both.

13. Evaluate the color, amount and consistency of the secretions and document the information on the patient's chart.

14. If further suctioning is necessary, use a fresh glove and sterile catheter.[3]

15. Administer oxygen before and after the procedure if ordered.

Oxygen Devices

When a patient has trouble breathing or has a low oxygen saturation level, oxygen may be ordered. This can be delivered via **nasal cannula** (a small plastic tubing that fits over the ears and has two prongs that fit into the nostrils through which oxygen is delivered; see photo below) or a mask that fits over the mouth and nose. The amount of oxygen to be delivered determines what device is used. Low levels of oxygen (2–6 liters per minute) can be delivered via nasal cannulas, moderate levels (5–10 liters per minute) are delivered via a simple facemask, and levels above 10 liters per minute are delivered via a reservoir or nonrebreathe mask (a mask similar to the simple facemask, but it also has a bag attached [the reservoir] that concentrates the oxygen and allows a higher level of oxygen to be delivered to the patient).[4]

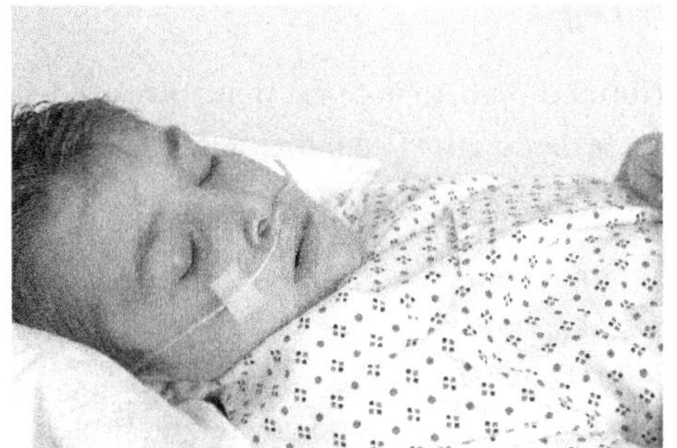

© Leah-Anne Thompson, 2013. Used under license from Shuttershock, Inc.

A simple facemask (below) is made of flexible plastic and fits over the patient's nose and mouth with elastic bands that go over the head to hold it in place.

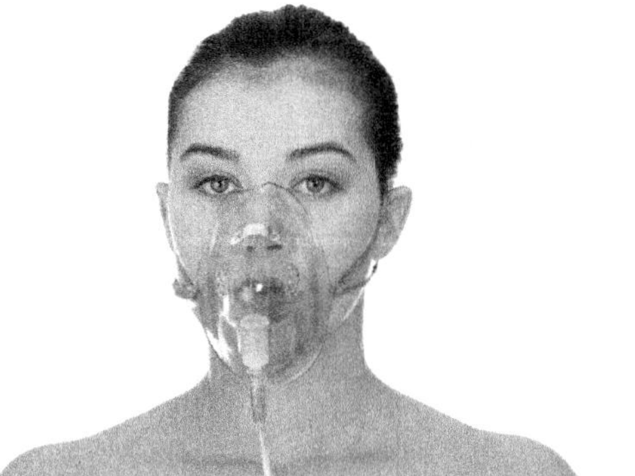

© Piotr Marcinski, 2013. Used under license from Shuttershock, Inc.

[3] Randle, Coffey & Bradbury (eds.). (2009). *Oxford handbook of clinical skills in adult nursing* (310). Oxford: Oxford University Press.

[4] www2.warwick.ac.uk/fac/med/research/hsri/emergencycare/prehospitalcare/jrcalcstakeholderwebsite/clinicalpracticeupdates/oxygen_guideline_combined_final_published_version_22apr09sb.pdf

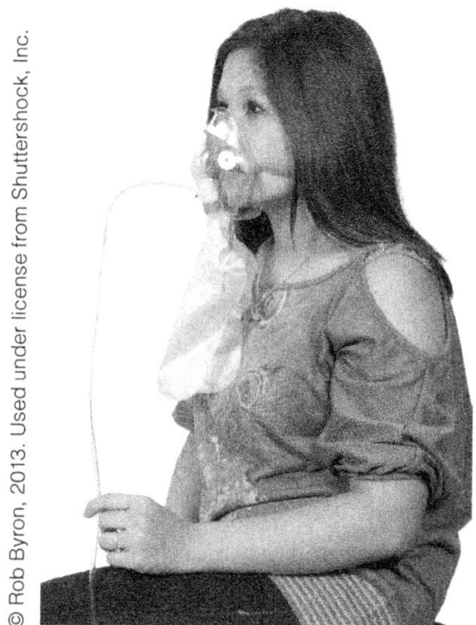

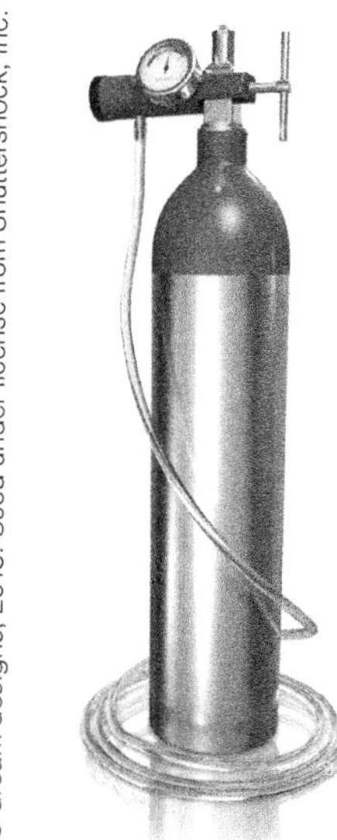

A reservoir, or nonrebreathe, mask (above)

The amount of oxygen to be delivered is determined by the patient's oxygen saturation. In a hospital, it is most likely that the oxygen supply comes from a supply piped into the patient rooms. In this case, the oxygen mask tubing is connected to the wall and the amount of oxygen delivered to the patient controlled with a flowmeter.

Oxygen is also delivered via oxygen tanks filled with compressed gas. When using an oxygen tank, you must be careful that the tank is kept upright and securely connected to a support frame.

Another option for outpatient use is an oxygen concentrator. This is a machine that removes nitrogen from the air, leaving almost pure oxygen.

When a hospital patient receives oxygen therapy, the oxygen supply most likely comes from the piped-in oxygen. However, when the patient needs to be moved to another location in the hospital, the oxygen supply needs to go along. This is done by switching the patient from the wall oxygen to a portable supply. Follow these steps to attach a patient to a green portable oxygen tanks:

1. Unscrew the top cover to expose thevalve.
2. Use the attached wrench to open the valve until you hear the hiss of released oxygen, then close the valve. This released oxygen blows any debris out of the connections that could harm the patient or the tank.
3. Apply the **regulator**, a device attached to the top of the tank that releases the oxygen at a predetermined rate. The regulator should fit over the top of the tank with two pins that fit into the tank.
4. Manually tighten the regulator. Using the wrench that you used to open the tank, tighten the regulator at least two full turns.

   If you hear or feel a leak, make sure the regulator is closed. If there is still a leak, close the tank and open the regulator and let the gas flow until the PSI (pressure per square inch) reads 0. Remove the regulator and try a different regulator.

5. Connect the patient's oxygen delivery device to the regulator. There may be a "Christmas tree" adaptor, which screws onto the regulator and allows the device tubing to quickly attach. If there is no adaptor, attach the tubing to the regulator.

6. Set the flow rate according to the physician's orders or to match the flowmeter on the wall oxygen.[5]

If the patient has a tracheotomy, there are special oxygen masks that can be attached to the opening of the tracheotomy tube. Oxygen is delivered through this tubing in the same manner as with nasal cannulas or facemask.

Drains

Following surgery a patient often has a drain inserted at the surgical site to assist with fluid removal, decompress air in the wound, and collect fluid to monitor healing. Surgical drains can be made of **silastic**™ (an artificial rubber) or rubber, can be open or closed, and can be active or passive. A **silastic**™ drain causes little tissue reaction; rubber drains can cause tissue reaction or the development of a tract (an opening from the skin to the area of surgery). An **open drain** dispels fluid onto a gauze pad or into a collection bag. This type of drain has a higher incidence of infection than does a **closed drain**, which drains into a bag or bottle. An **active drain** is attached to suction to move fluid into the collection site; a **passive drain** allows the fluid to drain according to differences in pressure between the inside of the body and the outside.

Leave the drain in place until fluid is no longer coming from the wound or less than 25 mL per day is produced. Drains in surgical sites can be left in place up to 7 days. The amount of fluid extracted helps determine the amount of fluid that needs to be replaced. This fluid can be saline or saline with electrolytes . Use standard precautions when dealing with patients with drains, keeping the area around the drain clean and the drain in the proper position without any kinks in the tubing. When removing the drain, the patient may experience some discomfort, but if the drain is removed before tissue grows around it, there should be little reaction afterward.[6]

S.K.I.L.L. Check

Which feeding tube doesn't gain access through the naso passageway?

Notes:

Tubes

Tubes are used to provide fluid management and drainage, provide nutrition, and monitor internal body functioning. Tubes are generally made from plastic or rubber and may have a single opening within the tube or multiple openings.[7] Some types of tubing are nasogastric, endotracheal, gastrostomy, and chest.

---

[5] web.missouri.edu/~danneckere/pt316/case/pulm/Strickland-bronchial_hygiene_for_PT-2009.pdf

[6] www.perspectivesinnursing.org/pdfs/Perspectives16.pdf

[7] www.globalspec.com/learnmore/flow_control_fluid_transfer/pipe_tubing_hose_fittings_accessories/medical_tubing

A **nasogastric** (**NG**) tube is inserted through a nostril and terminates in the stomach. This type of tube removes the stomach contents, which could be air or fluid. NG tubes deliver nutrients when the patient cannot take food or fluids by mouth. An NG tube can also remove stomach contents if a patient has ingested a poison or is vomiting blood.[8]

An **endotracheal** (**ET**) tube is similar to a nasogastric tube in that it is inserted into the nose but this tube is directed into the trachea. An ET tube delivers anesthesia during surgery, provides oxygen to a patient, and is used in procedures to examine the lungs.[9]

NG, NJ, ND, and PEG Tubes[10]

A **gastrostomy** (feeding) tube delivers nutrients to patients who cannot maintain their nutrition in a normal fashion. This tube can be inserted like a nasogastric tube or can be inserted via a puncture through the abdominal wall into the stomach.[11]

The insertion point of the feeding tube is indicated in abbreviation (NG) nasogastric, insertion place is through the (N) Nasal; with the tube end placement indicated in the last letter of the abbreviation (G) gastric. An (NJ) nasojejunal, (N) Nasal, (J) Jejunum, and a ND nasoduodenal tube is inserted at the (N) Nasal and placed in the (D) Duodenal area. The NG, NJ, and ND tubes are placed to provide nutrition and supplemental aid to patients who are unable to acquire adequate oral nutrition.

(PEG) tube stands for a Percutaneous Endoscopic Gastric Tube; a feeding tube that punctures through the external abdominal wall through to the stomach. This is done with the guidance of an endoscopic procedure for the tube placement. The PEG tube is a means of providing nutrition to patients who are unable to acquire adequate oral nutrition due to trauma, injury, paralysis, or other conditions that may prohibit regular means of oral nutrition.

A **chest tube** is inserted through the chest wall to remove air, fluids, or pus from the chest cavity. Air or fluids that are outside the lungs but in the chest cavity cause a pneumothorax (air in the chest cavity outside the lungs) or hemothorax (collection of blood in the chest cavity outside the lungs) and, therefore, breathing problems.[12]

Tube maintenance should follow universal precautions (see chapter 3 for an explanation of universal precautions), keeping the areas around the tubes clean and dry. Some tubes have balloons that are inflated to prevent the tube from moving farther into the patient or to prevent dislodgement.

Catheters

A **catheter** is a specialized tube used for a specific purpose, such as to administer medications directly into the body, measure the pressure inside an artery or vein, or remove fluids (serum, blood, pus) from a body cavity, to name a few uses. The care of catheters is the same as the care for tubes and drains.

---

[8] www.medterms.com/script/main/art.asp?articlekey=9349

[9] www.equipmentexplained.com/physics/airway/ett/endotracheal_tubes.html

[10] Jordan, R. (2013). Basic Client Care: Support Equipment [PowerPoint presentation and Lecture, Fall, 2013].

[11] www.nlm.nih.gov/medlineplus/ency/article/002937.htm

[12] lungcancer.about.com/od/glossary/f/chesttube.htm

Use the universal precautions when dealing with a patient who has a drain, tube, or catheter. Always wear gloves when administering care around the tube entry site. When transferring the patient, be aware of the tube location and ensure it is not kinked or dislodged during the move. Different tubes have different requirements as to how the the tube should be in relation to the patient to allow fluids to be withdrawn or inserted. Be sure you understand these requirements and follow them when working with the patient.

When providing patients with basic care, remember to always focus on the patient's needs. Use universal precautions when working with any equipment. Keeping the patient comfortable should be the focus of all care and treatment while in a hospital or care center.

SKILL Check Activity

Provide the Use

Divide the class into groups of various sizes and have them select the equipment for the other teams to define. Have the students then select ten pieces of support equipment from the text and ask each of the different groups to provide the parameters of the equipment use. This exercise familiarizes the students with the use of and the equipment variations. Note: if the instructor chooses, they may select a few to be used as bonus or tie breaking points.

Chapter 5 *Questions*

1. What are *physiologic needs*? Why are they important to know about?

2. You are working with a patient who cannot get out of bed. Describe the steps you would take to help the patient use a urinal.

3. What is an *emesis basin*? When would this be used?

4. Why would oral suctioning be necessary? How does this differ from nasal suctioning?

5. What is *CPR*? In a medical setting, who should know CPR?

6. You are helping a patient to the bathroom. On the way, the patient faints. What would you do to help the patient?

7. Why would skeletal traction be used? *- To keep bones in perfect alignment during healing phase*

8. A patient has a low oxygen saturation level, and the physician orders 8–10 liters of oxygen per minute for the patient. What type of equipment would be used to accomplish this?

O2 mask (5-10 ltrs) cann 2-6 ltrs Reserv = >10 ltrs

9. Why would a patient have a chest drain following cardiac surgery? How long would this type of drain be left in the patient's chest?

up to 7 days   oR <25 ml per day

10. Name four types of tubes and the purpose of each type.

NG Nasogastric Nostril → stomach remove air/vomit/blood
ET Endotracheal Nostril → trachea anestesia, O2 examine lungs

Gastronomy - NG, NJ, ND, PEG - feeding
Chest Tube - removes pus, air, blood outside of lungs. but in chest cavity

ET Tube
NG Tube

Reservior >10 liters O2
flow meter
Concentrator

Documentation

Part of patient care is documenting in the medical record what has occurred. The information in the record is critical for providing continuity of care. Each person who treats the patient documents what occurred so the next person who works with the patient has that record to provide continued treatment.

Medical Record

The **medical record** is the collection of the documents related to patient care. The record may reside in a doctor's office, clinic, or hospital. The physical or electronic copy of the medical record belongs to the hospital, doctor's office, or clinic, but the information in that record belongs to the patient.

This document is a case history of chronological written accounts of a patient's medical history, complaints, examinations, physician's physical findings, results of diagnostic tests, therapeutic procedures, treatments, medications, and resulting effects.

The recorded information belongs to the patient who has a right to view, limit disclosure (privacy), or request in writing a copy of the records for transfer. Though the medical record information is the property of the patient, the written or documented portion of the record are the under the custodial care of the healthcare provider. The provider has the legal rights (physical control) and duty to protect, house, preserve, utilize, maintain accuracy, and possibly disclose information recorded in the medical record; all of which are governed by specific federal and state laws and or acts. In accordance with the HITEC Act of 2009 (Section 164.524)[1], a patient has the right to have access and review the documents created by their doctor.[2]

Under special conditions, the provider may even deny the patient the availability of the record—usually when it is not in the best interest of the patient. This is, and possibly will remain, a major point of contention based on the situation and condition.

---

[1] http://www.gpo.gov/fdsys/pkg/CFR-2011-title45-vol1/pdf/CFR-2011-title45-vol1-sec164-524.pdf

[2] http://www.hipaasurvivalguide.com/hitech-act-summary.php

S.K.I.L.L. Check

What are two purposes for documentation?

Who owns the Medical Record?

Notes:

When entering information into the medical record, or charting, these items are to be included.

- patient name and identification number;
- date and time;
- observations;
- treatment given; and
- care provider signature.

It is important that each page in the record contain the patient name and identification number. This ensures that what is included in the record all belongs to the same patient.

Each entry into the record must include a date and time. It is important to know when certain things occur, such as medication administration. Without a date/time, the patient may be overmedicated or not get the proper dosages.

After each patient encounter, the person providing the care must document what occurred. This should include an assessment of the patient prior to the treatment and a description of what was done. The report needs to be concise, descriptive, and factual. For example, when the CNA obtains routine vital signs, the entry may look like this:

12/15/12 1000 Pt lying in Fowler's position. BP 140/80, HR 73, temp 99.2, RR 15, O2 sat 94%.
Mary Conner, CNA

This entry would be easy to understand and follow-up treatment could occur without difficulty. The physician may read this entry and decide the patient needs to be placed on supplemental oxygen due to the lower-than-normal oxygen saturation level and may order further blood testing to follow up on the elevated temperature.

Formatting

A common way to enter information is in the S–O–A–P format. The

S = subjective,
O = objective,
A = assessment
P = plan.

Subjective information is what the patient tells the healthcare worker. **Objective information** is what was found during the exam. **Assessment** is the healthcare worker's diagnosis of the situation. **Plan** is what treatment will be given, what follow-up is necessary, etc. A chart entry may look like this:

S   Stiff finger joints. Patient says more severe after sleeping or nonuse. Stopped drinking, some weight loss.

O   On exam there is swelling and pain around joints of fingers, symmetrical involvement. Blood pressure: 144/85. Pulse: 67. Weight: 178

    X-ray: Narrowed joint space, osteoporosis at joint. Uric acid: 4.2.

A   Rheumatoid arthritis

P   Aspirin 10 grains q.i.d., phenylbutazone 100 mg q.i.d. #28. Return: 1 month.[3]

When making entries in the chart, follow these procedure.

1. Ensure the right chart is used (right patient and right room/bed).
2. Use the correct form.
3. If using a paper chart, make entries in black ink only.
4. Use military time.
5. Be brief, concise, and factual.
6. Spell words correctly.
7. Use only hospital-approved abbreviations.
8. If using a paper chart, return the chart to the place it was found.

Military time is based on a 24-hour clock starting at midnight, which is 0000. This means that 1 p.m. is 1300 hours. Using this form ensures that the time noted in the chart is accurate and everyone is using the same time.

Table 6.1	Military Time		
0000	Midnight	1200	Noon
0100	1 a.m.	1300	1 p.m.
0200	2 a.m.	1400	2 p.m.
0300	3 a.m.	1500	3 p.m.
0400	4 a.m.	1600	4 p.m.
0500	5 a.m.	1700	5 p.m.
0600	6 a.m.	1800	6 p.m.
0700	7 a.m.	1900	7 p.m.
0800	8 a.m.	2000	8 p.m.
0900	9 a.m.	2100	9 p.m.
1000	10 a.m.	2200	10 p.m.
1100	11 a.m.	2300	11 p.m.

Each hospital is required to have a list of approved abbreviations. These are the only abbreviations that may be used in the chart. The Joint Commission, which evaluates and accredits hospitals, has a list of dangerous abbreviations that are *never* to be used in a medical chart. These are:

---

[3] Chart note obtained from Diehl. Medical transcription: Techniques and procedures, 7th ed. Philadelphia, 2011.

Table 6.2	Official Do Not Use List*	
Do Not Use	**Potential Problem**	**Use Instead**
U, u (unit)	Mistaken for 0 (zero), the number 4 (four) or cc	Write "unit"
IU (International Unit)	Mistaken for IV (intravenous) or the number 10 (ten)	Write "International Unit"
Q.D., QD, q.d., qd (daily) Q.O.D., QOD, q.o.d, qod (every other day)	Mistaken for each other Period after the Q mistaken for I and the O mistaken for I	Write "daily" Write "every other day"
Trailing zero (X.0 mg)** Lack of leading zero (.X mg)	Decimal point is missed	Write X mg Write 0.X mg
MS MSO4 and MgSO4	Can mean morphine sulfate or magnesium sulfate Confused for one another	Write "morphine sulfate" Write "magnesium sulfate"

* Applies to all orders and all medication-related documentation that is handwritten (including free-text computer entry) or on pre-printed forms

** **Exception:** A "trailing zero" may be used only when required to demonstrate the level of precision of the value being reported, such as for laboratory results, imaging studies that report lesion size, or catheter/tube sizes. It may not be used in medication orders or other medication-related documentation.

© The Joint Commission, 2014. Reprinted by permission.

Currently, this list of dangerous abbreviations does not apply to electronic records and CPOE (computerized physician order entry) systems but the Commission is studying this and may apply this list to those types of records also.[4]

Confidentiality/Security

HIPAA (Health Insurance Portability and Accountability Act) legislation was passed by Congress in 1996. This Federal law was enacted to:

- provide patients with the ability to maintain healthcare insurance when they change or lose jobs;
- reduce healthcare fraud and abuse;
- mandate industry-wide standards for healthcare information provided in an electronic fashion and
- protect the patient's healthcare information.

The last provision requires healthcare providers to have in place methods to protect patient health information (PHI) when it is transferred, received, handled, or shared. This protection applies to all forms of medical records: paper, electronic, and oral. Finally, only the minimum information necessary for continuity of care is to be shared.

---

[4] www.jointcommission.org/assets/1/18/Do_Not_Use_List.pdf

What this means to the healthcare worker working directly with the patient is that whatever treatment rendered to the patient is confidential. The information is to be included in the chart but not shared with anyone other than those treating the patient. Failure to follow the HIPAA rules can lead to civil and criminal penalties. For inadvertently sharing the PHI, the minimum penalty is $100 per violation up to a maximum penalty of $50,000 per violation. If PHI is intentionally shared, the minimum fine is $50,000 with an annual maximum of $1.5 million.[5] Patient information is not to be shared with anyone.

Medical charts have traditionally been kept in a paper form, with each patient having their own chart. In a hospital, the charts fill up many feet of shelving. Hospitals and clinics are converting to electronic records and doing away with the file shelves. As part of the American Recovery and Reinvestment Act of 2009, Congress passed the HITECH (Health Information Technology for Economic and Clinical Health) Act. Part of this act provides an incentive for hospitals, clinics, and doctor's offices to adopt electronic medical records. Because of the amount of patient health information that will be shared, the privacy and security protections under HIPAA have been expanded.[6] Also under the HITECH Act, the ability for patients to access their own record has been expanded to include electronic formats.

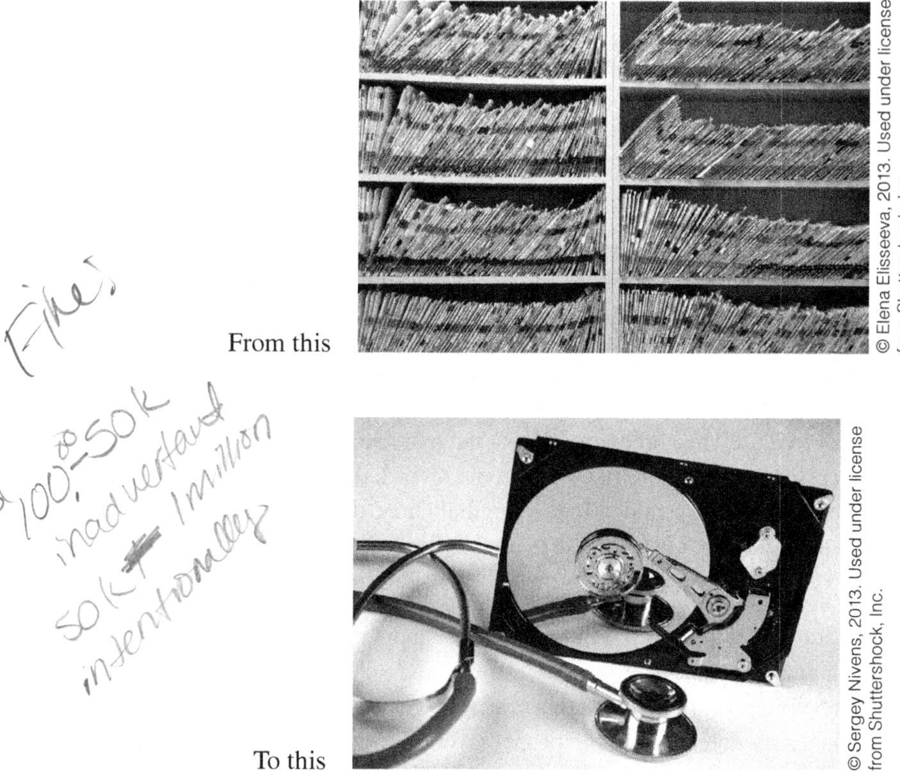

From this

© Elena Elisseeva, 2013. Used under license from Shutterstock, Inc.

To this

© Sergey Nivens, 2013. Used under license from Shutterstock, Inc.

---

[5] www.ama-assn.org/ama/pub/physician-resources/solutions-managing-your-practice/coding-billing-insurance/hipaahealth -insurance-portability-accountability-act/hipaa-violations-enforcement.page

[6] www.hipaasurvivalguide.com/hitech-act-summary.php

With the move to electronic records, charting is done differently. Instead of returning to a nursing station to find the chart, then finding the correct form, the healthcare worker uses a mobile computer station. The station is rolled to the patient room and information entered directly into the chart. The healthcare worker signs his or her entries electronically. This is done via software that requires the signer to enter a password to verify his or her name.[7]

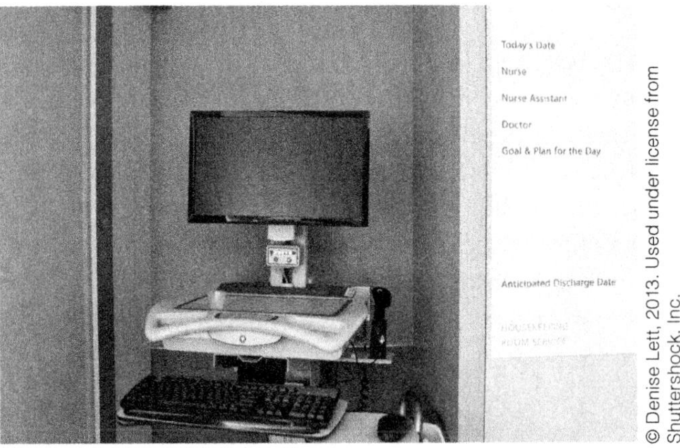

© Denise Lett, 2013. Used under license from Shuttershock, Inc.

The healthcare worker is also able to use a tablet or smart phone to make notes on patient care. However, these are not necessarily secure media and must used cautiously.

Oral documentation is also used, that is one healthcare worker verbally sharing patient information with another healthcare worker. One must be careful to share information in this manner with only the person who needs the information. Make sure the information is not shared in a busy hallway where other people may overhear.

Mistakes get made during charting. When this occurs, there are standard ways to fix the mistake. First of all, nothing may be erased or covered up. The author crosses out the mistake so it is still legible, initials the crossed out area, and adds the correct information. In an electronic record, the author makes an addendum to the original entry. The word "Addendum" is added to the original entry, the reason for the addendum is noted, the new entry is made, and the electronic signature is added. Sometimes an entry needs to be made out of time order. In this case, a "Late Entry" notation is made before entering the information.[8]

Never make an entry about a patient encounter or event before it has happened. Doing so may cause harm to the patient. For example, if a nurse is administering medications and notes in the chart that the patient received a dosage of Coumadin before giving it to the patient, but then gets called away and the patient does not get the medication, the patient may not maintain the proper level of drug in his or her system.

Medical records are not only for medical use; they are also considered legal documents. As such, the record can be subpoenaed in court. In the case of a malpractice suit against a physician, the medical record is a major part of the information provided for the case. Remember this when entering data into the record. Be sure it is accurate, the dates and times are correct, and the entry is signed properly.

---

[7] Gartee. Electronic health records: Understanding and using computerized medical records, 2nd ed. Prentiss Hall Publishing, 2011.

[8] http://www.ehow.com/how_6155952_make-corrections-electronic-medical-record.html

The medical record should contain certain information. A list of what is included in a medical record at the University of California hospitals includes: [9]

- patient name and address at time of admission;
- identification number (hospital number, Medicare number, Social Security number, or Medi-Cal number);
- age;
- sex;
- marital status;
- legal status;
- religious preference;
- admission and discharge dates;
- initial diagnostic impression;
- discharge diagnosis and disposition;
- advance directives;
- medical history;
- physical examination;
- consultation reports;
- order for medications, treatments, prescriptions, etc.;
- progress notes;
- nurses' notes;
- graphic and vital sign sheet;
- laboratory test results;
- x-ray examination results;
- consent forms;
- operative and procedure reports;
- pathology reports;
- discharge instructions;
- discharge summary; and
- telephone encounters.[10]

Documentation is a large part of providing patient care. Information obtained about a patient, patient treatment, and patient response to treatment are necessary to provide continuity of patient care and ensure proper patient care.

---

[9] This is an abbreviated list. For the entire list, see policy.ucop.edu/doc/1100168/LegalMedicalRecord, pp. 16–17.

[10] policy.ucop.edu/doc/1100168/LegalMedicalRecord

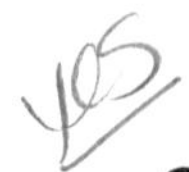

SKILL Check Activity

Patient Confidentiality

While working with another practitioner, you both pass an individual in the hall who stops the other practitioner and begins to ask questions about a client's condition and the procedure that you have just come from completing on the patient. You recognize the individual as a family member or close friend of the patient. The other practitioner explains the procedure and what its general purpose is and why it is used. The client's friend then goes on to ask what this means in relation to their friend's condition. The other practitioner elaborates on the generalized condition and what a test similar to what was done may contribute in information for a diagnosis and possible treatments. The practitioner does not mention the client's exact information or refer to the client during this portion of the discussion. After the brief discussion, the two of you return to your department to complete the paperwork and details. **Discuss:** With the class, what of this incident is considered appropriate and what may be considered a breach of confidentiality.

Chapter 6 *Questions*

1. Who owns patient medical records?

2. What is the purpose of a medical record?

3. What is to be included in an entry into a medical record?

4. Why are electronic records being used?

5. The clinic where you work uses electronic records. What would you do to ensure that an entry you make is in the correct record? What would you check to make sure you've got the right record?

6. It is change of shift and you are coming in to work in the assisted living center. A coworker is rushing around to get ready to leave and wants to give you updates about the patients you will be caring for. She is standing outside the patient rooms and rattling off information quickly. What would you do to make sure you got the information correctly and the information shared is kept confidential?

7. You have entered the information obtained when you took vital signs on a patient. As you were signing off on the entry, you realized that you had switched the temperature and pulse entries. What would you do to correct the entry?

8. What is a *SOAP note*? What do the letters stand for?

9. What is *military time*? Why is this format used in medical reports?

10. Patient records are used for continuity of patient medical care. What other uses might there be for the patient record?

Final-SO2?
Quizzes ////

BMI =
wght/hght 2

Personal Health and Common Conditions[1]

Personal Health

Health: The condition of the mind, body, and or emotions; moreover, the degree to which their state of being is free from illness or injury.

As healthcare practitioners we will see on a daily bases the choices that patients have made and the repercussions of some of those decisions. Many times, when looking after the health and wellbeing of others, we do not make the time or the effort to maintain our personal wellbeing. Being well is something that most people take for granted and something that does not necessarily come to mind, until it is in question.

By making a few solid choices in maintaining health, the risk of illness can be reduced. Through healthy eating habits, maintaining an ideal weight, resting, exercising, and maintaining healthy relationships; working in the healthcare facility and avoiding unnecessary stays in one is an achievable status. The last thing most people would want to see is someone with a runny nose, red eyes, and looking like they should be in the bed next to them standing over them.

Healthy Eating Habits

What to eat is a common topic to arise whether at home or out and about with friends. These choices and the decisions that are made are reflected in ourselves. Consider the decision to eat healthy an investment with a payoff that provides the opportunity to feel better and reduce the risk factors that can lead to a life of discomfort.

We have all heard the saying, "You are what you eat." Considering that the body repairs, fuels, and stores for future use what it is fed. How can the

<table>
<tr><td>

S.K.I.L.L. Check

Do you eat healthy?

Yes or No?

Name the food groups:

____

____

____

____

____

____

Notes:

</td></tr>
</table>

[1] Jordan, R. (2013). *Basic Client Care: Client and Personal Care* [PowerPoint presentation, Fall, 2013].

body make effective repairs and build with less than quality materials? Would a builder consider building their own home that they intended to stay in for any extended period or sleep soundly in, out of materials that were inferior? More than likely not, still look at the dietary choices that are made daily. Reflect on the desired outcome when it comes to how we keep ourselves healthier.

Eating healthy is something most have been exposed to since early childhood days. The basic food groups are: meats (beans, fish, and poultry, dairy); fruits; grains (bread and cereals); vegetables; and oils (fats and sweets to be used sparingly). By eating modest portions and exercising regularly, a person can support a longer healthier lifestyle.

Making small changes in our choices is the plausible and more effective way to adjust and maintain a course when it comes to a lifestyle change. Eating healthy is a choice and commitment to ourselves. The decision to improve our food choices is within our grasp and the choice is ours alone, as are the consequences of those decisions. Family health history and genetic dispositions are not within our power to change. Still, choices can be made to dissuade or enhance preventative measures to provide a better opportunity than the unknown alternative.

Maintain an Ideal Weight

It is not news that Americans are overweight with the majority at or past obesity. Knowing that excessive weight paves the way for obesity related conditions like high cholesterol, diabetes, high blood pressure, heart disease, stroke, depression, asthma, and some cancers—to name a few. The impact of weight reduces the opportunities of a longer healthier life span. Maintaining an ideal weight can be attained through eating healthy portions at meals and engaging in regular exercise.

Renew Energy

Many people can Identify with the all too familiar concept of being *dead on their feet*. When they go to bed they do not go to sleep, they lose consciousness. The average amount of required sleep, for most people, is six to eight hours; to recover, recharge, and repair from the period of being awake and surviving the rigors of daily work.

Rest is an important commodity that allows the mind and the body the time to breathe and relax. Breaks and lunch are allowed for this purpose, time to get away and allow for a refreshing minute to unwind. Taking a rest allows the mind a chance to regain focus and increase its ability to regain vitality. The ability to concentrate and listen with better acuity increases as does the ability to practice patience and tolerance. This is important in an atmosphere where tension and stress are a blended part of decision making. Consider rest recess for the mind.

Sleep is a necessity for the mind and body to recover, recharge, and repair. Sleep deprivation can have a serious impact on the ability to make decisions, reduce stress, and on the immune system. The benefits of sleep include: improved memory, weight control, enhanced mood, and improved health.

Exercise for Energy

Through regular exercise, we can maintain and create a baseline for personal health. The more sedate a personal routine becomes and stays, the less energy the subject has to effectively work with on a daily basis. A regular and intense exercise routine supports increased health, stamina, and energetic levels. Through regular exercise the maintenance of muscle and endurance can be increased and or sustained. Physical conditioning is the key factor in raising a person's energy levels and stamina; these factors are shaped by having the heart and lungs work more effectively and efficiently together during exercise.

The main two reasons most individuals do not exercise are that they do not have the time and they do not have the energy. Besides the benefits of increased health through exercise, the individual can gain energy and an improved mindset. Conditioning of the mind is as essential in our professional routine and in self-improvement. Exercise can create a healthy venue in which to review, resolve, vent, and express thoughts and problematic situations. Time is essential and a limited commodity for everyone, basically there are only twenty-four hours in the day. Effective and efficient time management is something all professional and successful individuals must learn to achieve.

Healthy Relationships

Healthy Relationships are built on quality communications between individuals. Relationships are the inevitability of living in a society of any size from a group of two persons to being an engaged global citizen. How relationships are maintained and supported reflect in our professional as well as in our personal lives. Benefits of healthy relationships can be mental wellness, improved immune system, stable support system, and the positive reinforcement of society. The basic elements of healthy personal and or professional relationships are: mutual respect, trust, personal responsibility, and open communication.

Stress and Stress Reduction

Stress: The body's response to internal unresolved conflict/forces.

Understanding what stress is helps us to identify the events, persons, situations, and ideals that make us susceptible to its effects. While providing professional care in the health service industry, providers are consistently exposed to stressful situations, elements, and persons. Long term exposure to stressful situations can cause harmful health effects to the provider. By identifying these factors, we can reduce stress by defusing and resolving the factors that may induce stress and its effects. Remembering that stress is individualized and personal to each person is helpful in considering the factors in its resolution.

What are some basic
elements of a healthy
relationship?

____

____

Name some stress
contributors:

____

____

____

____

Notes:

Stress Contributors

The following are examples of events or situations that cause stress and anxiety in people's lives daily. These factors have a significant impact due to intrinsic nature; these are things that we do not always control or have little ability to control though they can still majorly impact our lives. Planning and preparation are the best deterrents and resolving solutions for these

Example of Stress Contributors
- Serious Illness (self, loved one, relative, close friend)
- Death (self, loved one, relative, close friend)
- Financial Hardships (loss of job, unexpected bill, medical bill)
- Exams (school, work evaluations, medical tests)
- Relationships (divorce, domestic violence, arguments)

Identifying and Resolving

First, identify the stressor or more significantly why, what is present is stressful. Consider that most situations are temporary and that with time, the intensity will diminish. Look for plausible and reasonable solutions, if there are any. When a situation seems too large or complex to resolve with one solution; reassess to see if the situation can be segmented into smaller problems to be solved with possibly smaller solutions instead of one sweeping resolution. For stressful things that are unavoidable, it is best to have a plan of action that guides actions, reduces the amount of time in finding a course of action and may limit the exposure to the stressful event. Not all issues can be resolved quickly and easily; this is a process that is most effective when done thoroughly which may take time dependent on the degree of involvement of the stressor. Through repeated efforts in using this form of identifying and dealing with stressors, the practitioner will become more efficient and effective at resolving and dealing with stress and its effects.

When unavoidable events or situations occur, knowing how to reduce some of the factors to alleviate some of the symptoms may aid in diminishing the effects of stress on the individual. By emplacing and utilizing these stress reduction methods, stress can be diminished significantly. The following strategies have been used and have had varying degrees of success dependent on the individual:
- Breathe (a few slow deep breaths, allowing some tension to defuse)
- Be aware of mind, body, and emotional limitations
- Exercise regularly (mind and body)
- Rest (mind and body)
- Develop hobbies
- Develop a support system (family and friends)
- Take a break
- Prepare for unpleasant events
- Create balance in your life

- Develop your sense of humor
- Plan for what you can

Personal Time

Taking time to vacation, a short weekend trip, or just getting away from it all; is something that most professionals find hard to do. Using holiday and vacation time to recover from illness due to being run down from work or stress is not where or how that accumulated time is best spent. Personal time, hobbies, crafts, and activities are not simply diversions, they are time to get away and not be immersed in the work environment. This allotted time allows for the proverbial batteries to be recharged, breath of fresh air, and sanity break to occur. This gives the professional the opportunity to reset, rest and recuperate. These breaks allow for peak performance to be maintained, a reward for work well done. Remembering to reward your efforts and accomplishments is sacred ground to the wellbeing of the professional; we would like the Bahamas, but just getting away will do.

Common Conditions [2, 3, 4, 5, 6, 7, 8, 9, 10]

Within the healthcare spectrum, there may be some common occurrences t professionals will be exposed to with some frequency and from time to time. Due to the commonality of these, here are some basic points to become familiar with when involving these conditions.

In the following provided reading, some of the common conditions are listed with a broad definition which entails a basic understanding of the listing. A general description provides a brief medical explanation of the general complaint. Provided also are some of the signs and symptoms associated to offer a better understanding of the possible impact on the client and the considered care. The awareness segment is an initial reminder of how the healthcare practitioner may prepare to consider care. These are not diagnostic protocols, just delivery of care considerations.

---

[2] http://www.cdc.gov/

[3] http://www.nimh.nih.gov

[4] http://www.merriam-webster.com/dictionary/

[5] http://www.medterms.com

[6] http://www.oxforddictionaries.com

[7] http://health.utah.gov/epi/diseases

[8] http://www.rightdiagnosis.com

[9] http://www.who.int/en/

[10] http://www.news-medical.net

Client Distress

There are many things that may cause a patient distress while in a medical area. This can be anything from a splinter in an index finger all the way to respiratory arrest. The healthcare worker should be prepared to address anything that may be causing the problem.

All workers who come in contact with patients need to be certified in cardiopulmonary resuscitation (CPR). CPR classes including instruction on using an automatic cardiac defibrillator may be recommended and/or required by an employer.

The following are some items that may cause patient distress while in a hospital, with suggestions on treatment.

<u>Abrasion Definition:</u> This is a superficial wound caused by a scraping of the skin due to friction, grinding, and or rubbing.

> **Description:** This is a scrapped or worn area of skin due to friction, grinding, and or rubbing. With the resulting appearance of the affected area to be skinned and scrapped with the skin removed.

> **Signs and Symptoms:** This superficial wound may be painful, slightly swollen, red, oozing, with patchy or splotchy bleeding.

> **Awareness:** Be aware of injuries that the client has suffered particularly when moving, transporting, or assisting.

<u>Abuse Definition:</u> This is the systematic negative behavior in a relationship to gain and or maintain power/control over another. The directed behavior is expressed through mistreatment, cruelty, violence, intimidation, and or other negatively based reinforcers that are regularly repeated to achieve sustain control over another.

> **Description:** There are variations of abuse; the following are the most common:
> *Physical:* Through the use of; hitting, restraining, pushing, biting, kicking, punching, shaking, choking, and other harmful means.
> *Emotional:* Used to evoke negative and or helpless feelings in another by: cursing, blaming, swearing, attacks on self-esteem/belittling, criticizing the victim's thoughts and or feelings of worth.
> *Psychological:* Can be displayed through: threatening, throwing, smashing, breaking things, punching walls, hiding things, sabotaging situations and or possessions (car, computer, work environment, social interactions).
> *Sexual:* This can be any non-consenting sexual act, behavior, or contact.

> **Signs and Symptoms:** The victim may display various signs determined by the type of abuse they have been subjected to during the abuse cycle. Common signs are: fear, emotional numbness, low self-esteem, thinks they deserve the treatment, unexplained and or frequent bruising, and others again dependent on the type of abusive treatment.

> **Awareness:** As a healthcare practitioner, there is a duty to report any reasonable belief that abuse is occurring particularly if a minor or the elderly are involved. These rules may vary from state to state. It is always best to inform your supervisor or attending physician for a situational assessment.

Allergies Definition: This is a hypersensitivity that evokes an immune system response to a regularly harmless substance. The reaction may vary from discomfort to a severe reaction, up to and including death of the allergic subject. Again, the degree of the reaction may vary dependent on the susceptibility and tolerance ability of the client.

Description: There are primarily four ways a subject comes in contact with an allergen: airborne, ingested/food, injected, and contact with skin. *Airborne Allergens* can cause the sneezing, runny nose, itchy/bloodshot eyes and may cause irritation to the lung linings. Common sources include pet dander, pollen, and plant exposure. *Ingested/Food Allergens* can cause itching and swelling of the tongue, lips, and throat, while inducing nausea, vomiting, cramps, and diarrhea through the bowel tract, and may cause hives. *Injected Allergens* may be caused by injected medications, insect bites or stings. If the allergen enters the bloodstream, the result may cause a system-wide response also called anaphylactic shock. *Skin Contact Allergens* may cause a dermatitis which can involve reddening, itching, rash, and blistering.

Signs and Symptoms: These may vary dependent on the level of sensitivity and the amount of exposure to the allergenic material. Symptoms last from one hour to days following contact and may vary: pain, blistering, swelling, itchiness, hives, rashes, runny nose, cramping, and even death.

Awareness: This is the most common medical condition as there are an estimated 60 million plus Americans who suffer from allergies. The reaction may occur from within seconds to minutes of exposure to the allergen. Remember to check for possible allergies—with the patient, medical record, attending staff, the client indicators (medical alert tag or wrist band), as well as the patient room indicator for latex allergies.

Angina Definition: This is temporary chest pain and discomfort due to an insufficient amount of oxygen and or blood to the heart muscle.

Description: The pain and discomfort associated with angina has been described as severe pressure, squeezing, and crushing feeling accompanied with a suffocating sensation from just behind the breastbone.

Signs and Symptoms: Angina primary characteristic is pressing pain or sensation of heaviness. Additional signs and symptoms that the client may experience are pain in the shoulder, arm, neck, or jaw regions; nausea, fatigue, shortness of breath, diaphoresis, dizziness, and or weakness.

Awareness: There are several contributing factors that can promote angina: high emotional or psychological stress, extreme temperatures, heavy meals, smoking, and alcohol use can also cause or contribute to an onset of angina. Angina can be a precursor of a heart attack; all chest pain should be checked by a doctor. If chest pain persists longer than a few minutes and is not alleviated by rest it may be a sign of a heart attack. This is a medical emergency Call 9–1–1.

Asthma Definition: A respiratory condition that causes difficulty breathing through spasms and constriction of the bronchial airways.

Description: Clients complain of shortness of breath with tightness in the chest, coughing, and wheezing may be evidence of the condition.

Signs and Symptoms: Asthma signs and symptoms include:
- Shortness of breath
- Chest tightness or pain
- Coughing or wheezing
- A whistling sound may be present during exhalation.
- Coughing or wheezing attacks that are worsened by a respiratory viruses, such as a cold or the flu

Awareness: Asthma can't be cured, but its symptoms can be controlled. Because asthma often changes over time, clients with asthma may be susceptible to respiratory viruses, colds, or flus.

Contusion Definition: A bruising or injury to the skin from a blunt blow or crushing, the damage usually does not break the skin though it still ruptures the small blood vessels.

Description: Leaked blood from broken vessels, causing a blackish blue discoloration under the skin.

Signs and Symptoms: The contused or bruised area may be tender and or hot to touch, swollen, and may vary in color from a blue, purple, red, and yellowing dependent on the condition and age of the contusion.

Awareness: Understand that inadvertently touching or applying pressure may cause discomfort and pain to the client. This may also affect the patient's ability to move about.

Bronchitis Definition: Bronchitis is an inflammatory condition that involves the air passages leading and into the lungs; structures involved include the trachea, main stem bronchus, bronchi, and bronchioles.

Description: The bronchitis condition most commonly involves a productive cough and sputum. This may persist for months with the condition progressing and sputum production intensifying from clear to yellowish green, and may become blood shaded. There are two primary types of bronchitis—acute or chronic.

Signs and Symptoms: Acute bronchitis can typically initialize with generic common cold symptoms; runny nose, sneezing, and a cough. As the symptoms progress the cough becomes more painful, productive, (greenish, yellow phlegm/ sputum) with a fever, shortness of breath, and wheezing.

Awareness: Acute bronchitis can follow viral infections, which include common colds or influenza, which may still be followed by a secondary bacterial infection. Bronchitis is a primary concern when infants, young children, and the elderly are involved due to their weaker immune systems. In the instance of chronic bronchitis, the health practitioner must consider that it is a sign of serious lung disease that may be slowed but cannot be cured.

Cold Definition: Also called the common cold, this illness is a contagious, upper respiratory system, viral infection that includes the nose, throat, sinuses, eustachian tubes, trachea, larynx, bronchial tubes, and lung fields.

Description: The cold is a viral infection of the upper respiratory tract that may involve the nose, throat, sinuses, eustachian tubes, trachea, larynx, bronchial tubes, and lung fields. This upper respiratory infection reduces the ability to resist bacterial infections and creates favorable conditions for secondary infections to occur.

Signs and Symptoms: Common cold signs and symptoms present themselves in stages. Primary stages involve scratchy throat, runny nose, sneezing, and clear initial discharge. Secondary stages include yellowish green discharge, low fever, nasal congestion, headache, sore throat, fatigue, muscle aches, and lack of appetite. The illness may persist for up to three weeks with the cough remaining persistent.

Awareness: Most colds are contagious for the first week, approximately. The dominant modes of disease transmission for a cold are droplet and contact transmission. When an infected individual speaks, coughs, and or sneezes, contaminated droplets are expelled. The primary portal of entry is the respiratory system where the inhaled virus establishes in the nose and airways. If an individual makes contact with any infected surface (table, cup, computer, hand, etc.) the virus may be transferred to other uninfected individuals.

<u>Convulsions Definition:</u> This condition is an uncontrollable violent shaking of the body due to uncontrolled involuntary muscle contractions. Some neurological conditions may precipitate abnormal electrical activity in the brain with the resulting physical manifestations being convulsions, sensory disturbances, and or loss of consciousness.

Description: The body twitches, shakes, spasms, and or jerks involuntarily and uncontrollably due to abnormal health conditions or illness. Some noted conditions or illness that may contribute to this condition are seizures, fever, meningitis, hypoglycemia, head trauma, tumor, congenital or genetic defects, poisoning, drug, and or alcohol abuse.

Signs and Symptoms: Typical convulsion signs and symptoms may include muscle spasms, twitches, shakes, spasms, jerks, blackout, confusion, drooling, grunting or snorting, unusual rolling of the eyes, clenching or grinding of the teeth, loss of consciousness, loss of control of the bowel and of bladder functions are not uncommon.

Awareness: In the instances of seizures, occasionally convulsion may be preceded by nausea, anxiety, dizziness, and vision irregularities (spots, halos, flashing lights). For additional information, see seizures.

<u>Cyanosis Definition:</u> This is the bluish, grayish, or dark purple discoloration of the mucous membrane, skin, lips, nail bed, fingertips, and or toe tips due to insufficient oxygen.

Description: This bluish, grayish, or dark purple discoloration is caused by an oxygen insufficiency in the bloodstream. The capillaries in the skin and/or mucus membranes have an increased amount of carbon dioxide as well as the reduced oxygen.

Signs and Symptoms: Cyanosis is a physical sign of discoloration. The blue or purple discoloration of the skin or mucous is a sign of asphyxiation due to the insufficient oxygen levels in the blood.

Awareness: The pinkish coloration of the mucosal lining is due to the capillaries having proper oxygenation levels in the bloodstream. Blood that is rich in oxygen is bright red in color, whereas blood that is low in oxygen is darker. When looking for signs of cyanosis, inspect areas that have little pigment or melanin in them; some of the following areas are suggested due to the ample blood flow and capillary content: tongue, nail bed, lips, eye lids, finger tips, and toe tips.

Death Definition and Description: The end of life of a person or organism, a permanent cessation of vital functions.

Awareness: As a healthcare provider, this is an instance when being aware of the family's need for privacy, empathy, and care is the continued responsibility of the provider. There are grief counselors and personnel to see to the specific needs and process. Also consider the cultural concepts of the client and their family.

Dehydration Definition: The process of the removal of water/moisture, sodium, and electrolytes; this may impair the body's ability to perform regular functions. In severe cases dehydration is a medical concern.

Description: Loss of bodily fluids to the point that may impair function. The loss of fluids or dehydration can come from intense diarrhea, vomiting, fever, excessive sweating, or depravation of hydration.

Signs and Symptoms: Dehydration is likely to cause: dry mouth, thirst, sleepiness, lethargy, low urine output, dark urine, lightheadedness, headache, lack of sweating or tearing, confusion, sunken eyes, low blood pressure, fever, rapid breathing, and increased heart rate.

Awareness: Common causes of dehydration include: excessive sweating, diarrhea, fever, and vomiting. This condition can happen to anyone, although young children, the elderly, and some individuals with certain chronic illnesses are more susceptible.

Depression Definition: A mental illness that increases the feelings of despondency, dejection, and persistent sadness.

Description: The client suffers from severe despondency, dejection, loss of interest or interaction in day-to-day activities. The chronic feeling that life is not worth living coupled with persistent sadness and hopelessness presents a serious medical condition.

Signs and Symptoms: Clients who suffer from depression may have difficulty concentrating; feel fatigued; have difficulty with details and making decisions; experience loss of interest; feel sad, irritable, and frustratedhave reduced sex drive; sleep excessively or suffer from insomnia; go through crying spells;and they may have frequent thoughts of death, dying, or suicide.

Awareness: Be aware that depression affects people in different ways and can affect children and adolescents as well as adults. Sadness and unhappiness are considered normal temporary reactions to certain circumstances or situations; these conditions and depression differ in their duration and severity.

Diabetes Definition: A metabolic disease and condition that affects the body's ability to produce any or enough insulin.

Description: This chronic disease and condition affects how the body produces and or uses the glucose/sugar in the blood. In Diabetes Mellitus there are two primary conditions: Type 1 and Type 2 diabetes. Type 1: is when the body is no longer able to produce insulin and must receive insulin from an alternative source (insulin pump, or injection). Type 2: is a chronic lifelong condition where the body does not produce enough insulin to keep the blood glucose levels at a normal level. The third category is gestational diabetes which occurs during pregnancy, and usually resolves itself after the baby is delivered.

Signs and Symptoms: Common symptoms may :; excessive thirst, excessive hunger, increased urination, unusual weight loss or gain, extreme fatigue, blurry vision, slow healing, tingling, pain, agitation, and or altered level of consciousness.

Awareness: Onset of diabetes can occur at any age; risk factors in increasing the chances of prediabetes are obesity, inactivity, family history, race, high blood pressure, and age. There are additional factors that may also contribute to Type1, 2, and or gestational diabetes.

<u>Diaphoresis Definition:</u> This is perceptible and profuse sweating.

Description: The excessive sweat secretions are usually associated with physical exertion, exposure to increased heat, mental and or emotional stress. In many cases, diaphoresis may have several causes associated with it—other conditions, disease, injury, and or illnesses.

Signs and Symptoms: Diaphoresis is a non-specific or general sign, which means that it may have many possible causes.

Awareness: A client displaying this condition may be self-conscious of and sensitive to their excessive exocrine secretions. The healthcare professional must be aware when considering the social impact and possible apprehension and or embarrassment of the client when interacting with personnel.

<u>Domestic Violence Definition:</u> Abusive behavior used by persons in a relationship in relation to establishing control over one partner in the relationship.

Description: Partners in the relationship may be married or not; heterosexual, gay, or lesbian; living together, separated or dating. There are variations of abuse; the following are the most common:
Physical: Through: hitting, restraining, pushing, biting, kicking, punching, shaking, choking, and other harmful means. Emotional: Used to evoke negative and or helpless feelings in another by: cursing, blaming, swearing, attacks on self-esteem/belittling, criticizing the victim's thoughts and or feelings of worth.
Psychological: Can be displayed through: threatening, throwing, smashing, breaking things, punching walls, hiding things, sabotaging situations and or possessions (car, computer, work environment, social personal and professional interactions).
Sexual: This can be any non-consenting sexual act, behavior, or contact.

Signs and Symptoms: The victim may display various signs determined by the type of abuse they have been subjected to during the abuse cycle. Common signs are: fear, emotional numbness, low self-esteem, thinks they deserve the treatment, unexplained and or frequent bruising, and others, again dependent on the type of abusive treatment.

Awareness: As a healthcare practitioner, there is a duty to report any reasonable belief that abuse is occurring, particularly if a minor or the elderly are involved. These rules may vary from state to state. It is always best to inform your supervisor or attending physician for a situational assessment. Domestic violence and emotional abuse are behaviors used by one person in a relationship to control the other. Partners may be married or not married; heterosexual, gay, or lesbian; living together, separated or dating.

Dyspnea Definition: This condition is the uncomfortable awareness of having the urge to breathe, a difficulty with breathing, or shortness of breath; it is caused or aggravated by lack of oxygenation of the bloodstream.

Description: This is usually described as an intense sensation of suffocation accompanied with tightening and heaviness of the chest; it has also been described as air hunger.

Signs and Symptoms: An individual may experience some or all of the following signs and symptoms. A noticeable labored breathing pattern in conjunction with anxiety, flaring nostrils, gasping, cyanosis, fatigue, and distressed expressions are the more common developments.

Awareness: Dyspnea may represent a disease of the lungs (asthma, pneumonia, COPD, congestive heart failure, and or ischemia). Other conditions have been known to aggravate Dyspnea such as: massive obesity, high altitude, extreme temperature, or over strenuous activity.

Edema Definition: The excessive accumulation of fluids in the soft tissues, which results in swelling due to an abnormally increased volume of serous fluid.

Description: Edema is primarily characterized by swelling of the tissues due to serous fluid leakage from the circulatory system and then the accumulated fluid remains in the tissue spaces and or body cavity. In the instance and imbalance of edema, the normal transport and absorption of serous fluid is compromised or precipitated by trauma, illness, injury, disease, and or other conditions that result in swelling.

Signs and Symptoms: Edema is a sign that is emphasized by puffiness and stretched appearance of the skin. When the skin is pressed, it can be painful and will remain dimpled for several seconds or longer. In relation to pulmonary edema, the client will likely have difficulty breathing, shortness of breath, congestion, wheezing, chest pain and or a wet cough that is productive.

Awareness: In most instances of injury or reaction, edema is a normal response to such occurrences. Direct trauma due to a sprained ankle or wrist or a reaction to an animal or insect sting or bite may also produce an inflammatory response. In severe instances, swelling can become a danger to the client—particularly involving respiratory responses. These may be initiated by any of the aforementioned circumstances and edema can be a result of medical conditions or allergenic reactions to medications, foods, or substances.

Febrile/Fever Definition: This condition is usually indicated by the presence of an abnormally high body temperature (100 degrees or higher) in a subject.

Description: The presence of a fever or a temperature above the acceptable normal variation of 99 degrees. High fevers over 103 degrees may cause additional, more serious signs and symptoms. Over an extended period, these higher temperatures may cause permanent brain damage.

Signs and Symptoms: The following may be an indication of fever: sweats, chills, chattering teeth, nausea, headache, hallucinations, confusion, weakness, convulsions, shivering, loss of appetite, and possibly dehydration.

Awareness: The presence of a fever may be an indicator of: pathogenic infection, inflammatory condition, trauma, malignancy, or drug side effect. Fevers in children and the elderly may be of particular concern because of their susceptibility to the extreme conditions. In infants, particularly with fevers over 101 degrees, a physician should be consulted.

Fracture Definition: A disruption or break in the continuity of the boney tissues and or cartilaginous structures.

Description: The disruption or break in the boney structure varies in degrees and are identified through different classifications including: **simple, compound, incomplete** and **complete**. A *simple* or *non-displaced fracture* is a break in the bone where the bone remains aligned. *Compound fractures* are distinguished by the characteristic of the broken bone fragments protruding through the skin, resulting in an open wound. An *incomplete fracture* or *green stick fracture* indicates that the bone break does not traverse completely through the bone. Whereas with a *complete fracture* the fracture has traversed completely through the bone and the fracture site may be complicated by displacing the fractured segments (the bone segments are apart). Note: A dislocation is indicated when the bony structures of any joint are displaced from their associated joint.

Signs and Symptoms: Symptoms may include swelling, disfigurement, redness, bruising, stiffness, and or immobility of the area of interest.

Awareness: Clients at a higher risk of fractures are usually in the following categories: persons engaged in high activity (children, athletes, and occupational hazards); elderly (due to loss of bone density); and persons with specific disease processes (osteogenesis, osteoporosis, cancer, tumors, and other degenerative processes). A radiograph is usually used to confirm the diagnosis.

Headache Definition: This is simply, pain in the head.

Description: Pain in the head that may vary in degrees of intensity, frequency, and duration. The pain may originate from a single or multiple reasons. There are a variety of types of headaches; some of the following are more common: episodic tension headaches, chronic tension headaches, migraine, cluster, and a variety of others.

Signs and Symptoms: Some of these may include: dull, aching head pain; increased sensitivity to either light or sound; a sensation of tightness or pressure across the forehead or on the sides and back of the head; tenderness on your scalp, neck and or shoulder muscles.

Awareness: Headaches are common, though their severity may vary from client to client. Studies have indicated that more than 90% of the female population and 70% of men have experienced some type of tension headache.

Hypertension Definition: This is a condition where the pressure of the blood flowing through the arteries of the body is higher than it should regularly be.

Description: A condition where the blood pressure is persistently elevated above the normal region. The ranges of blood pressure are considered the following: *Normal:* Systolic is below 120 mm Hg and Diastolic is less than 80 mm Hg; *Prehypertension:* Systolic range is 120–139 mm Hg and the Diastolic range is 80–89 mm Hg; *Hypertension Stage 1:* Systolic range is 140–159 mm Hg and the Diastolic range is 90–99 mm Hg; *Hypertension Stage 2:* Systolic range is 160 mm Hg or higher and the Diastolic range 100 mm Hg or higher.

Signs and Symptoms: For most people, there are little to no signs until the pressure begins to reach the severe region; some symptoms that may occur in clients with high blood pressure are: dull headache, trouble with memory or understanding, dizzy spells, blurred vision, and chest pain.

Awareness: Be aware that in most cases, people do not have any signs or symptoms and the condition can go on for years without discovery. The additional danger is that the body and its systems can be damaged by prolonged exposure to elevated pressures. Some of the possible complications may be: heart failure, aneurysms, arteriostenosis, heart attack, stroke, and possible metabolic disorders.

<u>Infection Definition</u>: An invasion or compromise of tissues with the multiplication of an invading pathogenic organism.

Description: The invading pathogen, by compromising the host, precipitates the Chain of Infection where the pathogen causes a progression of cellular failure, tissue failure, organ failure, system failure, and the eventual cessation of biological functions of the host organism.

Signs and Symptoms: These may vary and may be dependent on the type of pathogen, mode of transmission, and the portal of entry. General signs of a compromised host may be: fever, loss of appetite, nausea, vomiting, and muscle aches.

Awareness: Hand washing is the major preventative measure in fighting the spread of infection.

<u>Influenza Definition</u>: This is an acute, highly infectious respiratory and intestinal viral disease, commonly known as flu.

Description: This disease is classified primarily as a respiratory illness that produces a host of signs and symptoms (see below). The current influenza types are: A, B, and C; with each having degrees and or subtypes. Influenza types A and B are considered implicated in epidemic human disease. There is also the categorization of the viral structures (HN) subtype designations of which there are presently 16 H subtypes and 9 N subtypes.

Signs and Symptoms: The commonly characterized signs and symptoms may range from: body aches, fever (chills), lack of energy, muscle aches, dry cough, runny nose, sore throat, vomiting, and possibly diarrhea.

Awareness: Complications may arise from the aggravated instance of flu in conjunction with other known conditions and or illnesses including: pneumonia, bronchitis, infections, congestive heart failure, and asthma. Flu can create serious issues for infants, young children, pregnant women, and the elderly (those over 65).

<u>Laceration Definition</u>: A deep cut, tear, split, or gash in the skin as a result of an injury.

Description: These can be an irregular break in the skin and fall under five general classifications. *Split Laceration:* may occur when part of the body is crushed between two objects, or similarly when a blunt impact causes the skin to tear away. Split lacerations most commonly show up on the face, head, hands and legs. *Over-Stretching:* This wound would typically be the result of a unidirectional angled pressure that may push or pull the skin causing it to tear in a flap. *Grinding Compression/Avulsion:* An object strikes with a blunt impact at a sweeping motion or angle;the resulting wound is a grinding compression that peels away the top layer of skin. *Cut Laceration:* This wound is the likely result of a blade or sharpened object coming into contact with the skin with enough pressure to break the skin and tissues below.

This is the most common type of laceration. *Tearing:* A laceration of this type is the common effect of pressures from two directions applied to the skin and it is simply ripped or flayed open.

Signs and Symptoms: Dependent on the depth of the laceration, there can be a varied amount of bleeding, swelling and pain.

Awareness: The depth of wound and bleeding amount would dictate the amount of medical intervention, particularly in arresting the deeper wounds that have heavier bleeding. Cleaning and wound care are highly important to reduce the chances of infection due to the integumentary system being compromised.

Myocardial Infarction (Heart Attack) Definition: The death of heart muscle due to interrupted blood flow and or fatal interruption of the heart's normal functioning.

Description: A heart attack is a result of interrupted blood flow to the heart, which can damage or destroy the heart muscle. When the blood flow to a part of the heart is blocked for a long enough period of time, the part of the heart muscle that is deprived becomes damaged or dies. Usually, this occurs when an occlusion, blood clot, or severe stenosis blocks the flow of blood through a coronary artery.

Signs and Symptoms: A client experiencing a myocardial infraction may exhibit angina, chest tightness, left arm pain, dyspnea, light headedness, orthopnea, jaw pain, diaphoresis, nausea, or vomiting.

Awareness: A heart attack can also be caused by electrical disturbance or poor nerve conduction. Immediate medical and or CPR intervention in most instances is required for the victim to survive the incident or to recover. Treatment may vary dependent on the determination and origination of condition, based on qualified medical personnel determination, a best course of treatment will ensue.

Nausea Definition: An uneasiness or queasiness of the stomach; also an urge to vomit.

Description: The feeling of being sick to the stomach, queasy, or the increasing urge to vomit is identifiably marked as an unpleasant sensation preceding actual vomiting.

Signs and Symptoms: Nausea in itself is a symptom, though it may be accompanied by other parasympathetic signs or indicators; bradycardia, diaphoresis, paleness, and or salivation.

Awareness: Nausea may be present without actually vomiting. Vomiting may relieve the nausea sensation. Nausea is considered a general or nonspecific symptom that may be present due to illness, injury, psychological, emotional, and or physical stress.

Obesity Definition: This is the condition characterized by gaining excessive weight and retaining the overweight condition.

Description: The excessive amount of stored fat is not only a cosmetic concern but a health risk that increases risk factors for immediate and long term effects. The excessive weight gain and fat accumulation are presently measured and determined through a formula that considers a person's height and weight called Body Mass Index (BMI).

Signs and Symptoms: The signs and symptoms include excessive amounts of fatty tissue and increased BMI and waist circumference. Increased weight to the point of obesity can introduce weight related conditions, including: shortness of breath, joint pain, increased blood pressure, excessive sweating, and back pain.

Awareness: Health conditions that may accompany or become introduced through obesity include: high cholesterol (including high triglyceride levels), diabetes, high blood pressure, heart disease, stroke, sleep apnea, osteoarthritis, gallstones, depression, asthma, and some cancers.

<u>Post-Traumatic Stress Disorder (PTSD) Definition:</u> This is a mental health condition brought on by an excessively disturbing event that impacts the participant or observer.

Description: The psychological disorder that develops after a terrifying ordeal and involves the fight or flight response that becomes damaged, leaving the individual feeling stressed or frightened, even when the threat or danger is not present. The symptoms and distress may be re-experienced by the affected individual at the introduction of a trigger (an object, image, or event) that reminds the person of the situation.

Signs and Symptoms: These are a few of the commonly described signs and symptoms: re-experiencing spontaneous vivid memories of the traumatic event, avoidance, negative thoughts and temperament, loss of interest in activities, and arousal. An arousal could manifest in aggression, hyper vigilance, self-destructive behavior, recklessness, or fight response.

Awareness: Being afraid is a normal feeling for an individual in danger. Being mindful of a client's history of possible trauma; assaults, MVA, domestic violence, or survival of a military conflict could be helpful in diagnosis and treatment. For treatment consideration, a qualified mental health clinician and or personnel are recommended.

<u>Respiratory Distress Definition:</u> This condition is characterized as difficulty, labored, or pain with breathing.

Description: A condition usually indicated by difficulty, labored, or pain with breathing, which can be the result of disease, trauma, illness, or psychological experience; even with no physiological basis. The condition can affect the ability to exchange oxygen for patients with lung disease.

Signs and Symptoms: These signs and symptoms may vary dependent on the severity of the condition; the following are common with this condition: cyanosis, tachypnea (rapid breathing), rapid pulse (tachycardia), pulmonary edema, breathlessness, dyspnea, confusion, and extreme fatigue.

Awareness: In order to recover, a patient must receive a correct diagnosis of the underlying condition for accurate and proper treatment of this condition.

<u>Seizures</u>[11] **Definition:** This condition is abnormal electrical activity in the brain with the physical manifestations of convulsions, sensory disturbances, and or loss of consciousness.

Description: This condition of abnormal uncontrolled electrical activity in the brain, which may produce physical convulsions, slight physical signs, confusion, or a combination of symptoms. Seizures have two major classifications: Focal Seizures and Generalized Seizures; within these two primary classifications there are several additional categories. Focal Seizures involve one area of the brain where the abnormal activity persists. Three select categories within this classification include simple focal seizures, simple partial seizures, and dyscognitive focal seizures. In the classification of generalized seizures ,which entail seizures that all areas of the brain are involved, there are six additional categories. The categories considered amongst generalized seizures are: absence seizures (petit mal), tonic seizures,

---

[11] http://medical-dictionary.thefreedictionary.com/

clonic seizures, myoclonic seizures, complex partial seizures, atonic seizures, and tonic-clonic seizures (grand mal).

Signs and Symptoms: The signs and symptoms may vary dependent on the type of seizure involved. *Absence or petite mal seizures* are momentary lapses in consciousness and activity. The patient may develop a blank stare, lip smacking, fluttering eyelids, chewing motions of the mouth and/or small hand movements. Recovery is almost instantaneous and the patient has no memory of the episode.[12] *A tonic-clonic or grand mal seizure.* is the type seen in a patient with epilepsy. The patient will develop involuntary muscle contractions and stop breathing. The muscles will contract and relax in a repetitious manner. The patient may clench their teeth, bite their tongue, and lose control of bowel or bladder. After these symptoms abate, the patient may fall asleep or experience confusion, and when waking, won't remember the incident.[13]

Awareness: A febrile seizure is a convulsion particular in young children of seven years or under; that may be caused by a spike in body temperature, or often from an infection. Seizures include convulsions.

<u>**Sexually Transmitted Infections (STI/STD) Definition:**</u> A various number of diseases that are primarily contracted through sexual intercourse and or other intimate sexual contact.

Description: These infectious transmitted diseases may pass from person to person through blood, semen, or vaginal and other bodily fluids and or materials. Spread primarily through sexual intercourse and or other intimate sexual contact, these communicable pathogens infect a susceptible host with bacteria, parasites, and or viruses. There are more than 30 different types of infections in this STI/STD classification.

Signs and Symptoms: These may be dependent on the type and stage of the disease in which the host is infected; the signs and symptoms that might indicate an STI/STD presence include:
- Blisters
- Sores or bumps on the genitals or in the oral or rectal area
- Painful or burning urination
- Lesions
- Ulcers
- Discharge from the penis
- Vaginal discharge
- Discharge is odorous
- Unusual vaginal bleeding
- Sore, swollen lymph nodes
- Lower abdominal pain
- Rash

Awareness: Some such infections can also be transmitted nonsexually; instances of this include: from infected mother to infant during pregnancy or childbirth, blood transfusions, or shared needles (IV drug use, tattoos, piercings, etc.)

---

[12] http://reference.medscape.com/article/1183858-overview

[13] http://emedicine.medscape.com/article/1184846-overview

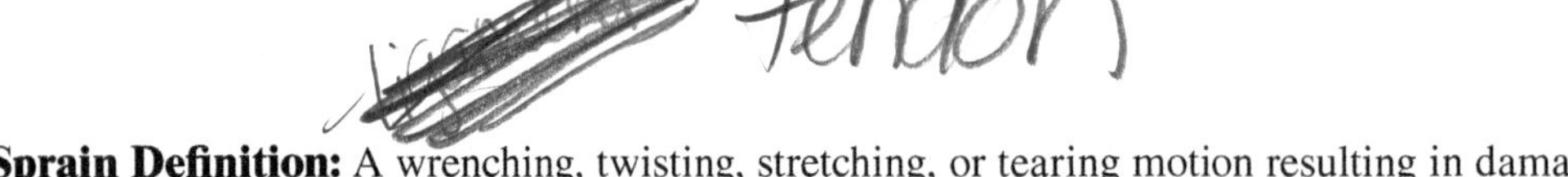

<u>Sprain Definition:</u> A wrenching, twisting, stretching, or tearing motion resulting in damage or injury to the tendon or fibrous connective tissues involved.

Description: This wrenching, twisting, stretching, or tearing motion subjects a joint to more physical force than it is structured to tolerate. The resulting injury can vary from First Degree to Third Degree. The degrees of injury are described as follows: *First Degree:* This is characterized by a stretching of the tissue involved without tearing of the fibers. *Second Degree:* This is characterized by the stretching and partial tearing of the involved fibers. *Third Degree:* This injury is characterized by the complete tear/separation or rupture from the structure.

Signs and Symptoms: The resulting injury can produce a variety of signs and symptoms dependent on the characterization of the injury. Some of these may be: bruising, pain, and swelling—ranging from mild to severe; this in conjunction with temporary to severe dysfunction of the part involved.

Awareness: Due to the structures involved, a radiograph may be required to rule out a possible fracture of the parts involved. Consider the client's comfort by minimizing use and movement while assisting transportation or by providing appropriate support.

<u>Strain Definition:</u> A wrenching, twisting, stretching, or tearing motion resulting in damage or injury done to the muscular tissues involved.

Description: This wrenching, twisting, stretching, or tearing motion subjects a joint to more physical force than it is structured to tolerate. The resulting injury can vary from First Degree to Third Degree. The degrees of injury are described as follows: *First Degree:* This is characterized by a stretching of the tissue involved without tearing of the fibers. *Second Degree:* This is characterized by the stretching and partial tearing of the involved fibers. *Third Degree:* This injury is characterized by the complete tear/separation or rupture from the structure.

Signs and Symptoms: The resulting injury can produce a variety of signs and symptoms dependent on the characterization of the injury. Some of these may be: bruising, pain, and swelling—ranging from mild to severe; this in conjunction with temporary to severe dysfunction of the part involved.

Awareness: Due to the structures involved, a radiograph may be required to rule out a possible fracture of the parts involved. Consider the client's comfort by minimizing use and movement while assisting transportation or by providing appropriate support.

<u>Stroke Definition:</u> This is a sudden blockage, interruption, or rupture of a blood vessel that results in the sudden death of brain cells due to lack of oxygen.

Description: This condition is the stoppage and or interruption of blood flow to brain often resulting in one or more of the following: facial drooping, loss of consciousness, weakness, paralysis, altered level of conscious, partial loss of movement, numbness, and or slurred speech.

Signs and Symptoms: The condition may induce some of the following results: facial drooping, loss of consciousness, weakness, paralysis, altered level of conscious, partial loss of movement, vertigo, confusion, inability to comprehend (speech, writing), numbness, and or slurred speech. There are two stroke categories; Ischemic Stroke and Hemorrhagic Stroke. An *Ischemic Stroke* is caused by thrombotic (blood clot) or embolic (cholesterol plaque) occlusion of an artery interrupting the flow of blood to the brain. While a

Hemorrhagic Stroke is the result of a weakened vessel that ruptures and bleeds into the surrounding brain tissue. The leaked blood accumulates and compresses the surrounding brain tissue causing it to expire.

Awareness: Medical intervention is critical within the first hour of the onset of signs and symptoms to have an accurate diagnosis for an attempt to save as much of the distressed or effected brain tissue or before the event can precipitate further. This is also known as cerebrovascular accident or CVA. The National Stroke Association has developed the acronym F.A.S.T., Face: Ask client to smile; Arms: Ask client to raise arms; Speech: Ask client to speak a simple phrase; Time: If any of the signs or symptoms are present call 911 immediately.[14]

<u>Trauma Definition:</u> A deeply disturbing event or serious injury to an individual from an incident involving violence or an accident producing shock to the body.

Description: The result of this extraordinary event in which serious injury or emotional wounding occurs creates substantial lasting psychological and or physical effects. The two primary types of trauma are psychological and physical trauma, of which can invoke a neurosis in the individual involved or witnessing the event. *Psychological Trauma:* This is an emotional response to a direct or indirect personal experience of an event that involves actual or threatened circumstance of death, physical integrity, and or serious injury of oneself or others; with the response of intense fear, helplessness, or horror. *Physical Trauma:* This is characterized by a physiological wound or injury caused primarily by an external source. The physical harm inflicted can vary from minimal to severe but still having psychological ramifications due to the situation, severity, or possible lasting physical effects, through anticipation or perception of the event.

Signs and Symptoms: These can vary dependent on the type and severity of the event. Psychological trauma may precipitate physical effects: insomnia, fatigue, muscle tension, agitation, aches and pains.

Awareness: Victims of trauma may respond differently to the event, circumstances, and treatment. Denial of complications in dealing with the event and or emotions is not uncommon for those involved.

<u>Traction Definition:</u> This is the utilization of pulling tension to treat muscle and skeleton disorders.

Description: Through pulling tension with traction devices and support equipment to treat muscle and skeleton disorders, these are used to align body structures for immobilization and treatment. There are two primary forms of traction. *Skeletal Traction:* This is a method of drawing, pulling, or extending with a pin or wire surgically inserted into an affected bone to immobilize, position, and align a fractured bone or structure properly and to facilitate the healing process. *Skin Traction:* This is a method of drawing, pulling, or extending through a mechanism consisting of adhesive or nonadhesive strapping attached to the skin surrounding the structure or limb to immobilize, position, and or align a structure properly and to facilitate the healing process.

Signs and Symptoms: Traction may be used to alleviate some signs and symptoms of the treated fractures primarily the following: pressure, pain, and muscle spasms.

Awareness: Before transporting or moving a client in this treatment format, have assistance and be cognizant of the weights and lines involved. Additional concerns for skeletal traction include the increased risk of infection at the pin insertion site and tract.

---

[14] http://www.stroke.org/site/PageServer?pagename=symp

<u>**Vomiting Definition:**</u> This is the voluntary or involuntary evacuation of the contents of the stomach through the oropharynx and or nasopharynx passageway(s); also known as throwing up.

Description: The heaving and or retching action of the stomach is a forceful expulsion of its contents in concert with a series of parasympathetic and sympathetic systems causing sweating and palpitations. An activated vomiting center of the brain stimulates increased salivation, deep breathing, and relaxation of the pyloric sphincter. An increase in abdominal pressure while simultaneously lowering of thoracic pressures assists in the ejection of the contents through the abdominal muscle contractions.

Signs and Symptoms: Vomiting itself is considered a sign and is commonly accompanied by increased sweating, palpitations, salivation, and deep breathing.

Awareness: A primary concern of excessive vomiting is dehydration. Rarely, excessive vomiting can induce a tear or rupture in the esophageal lining. A rupture of the esophagus is a medical emergency.

SKILL Check Activities

Personal Nutritional Review

Instructions: Considering the schedule most people keep and understanding the value of a nutritional meal, take the time to note for three days during the work/school week what and when you eat something. If there is someone present while eating, who is it? Chart out your eating habits for the three days and bring it in to class.

Key Information Memory (K.I.M.)

Use this graphic organizer to consolidate information and provide an easier way to relate the vocabulary with a definition by using a visual aid in a more familiar context to help identify the subject, definition, and concept. By placing the vocabulary word in one column, then writing the definition in the next, the user selects a memory cue to draw in the third column.

Questionnaire

1. How many meals a day do you eat?

2. Do you eat breakfast?
   a. If so, what does it consist of?

   b. What time do you eat?

3. Do you eat lunch?
   a. If so, what does it consist of?

   b. What time do you eat?

4. Do you eat dinner?
   a. If so, what does it consist of?

   b. What time do you eat?

5. Do you eat your meals alone or with others?
   a. If so, with whom?

6. Do you think you have good eating habits?

7. Do you exercise? If so, how often?

Chapter 7 *Questions*

1. How does weight change our life style?
   a. Less activity:

   b. Energy:

   c. Decreased lifespan:

2. Does a diet effectively work?
   a. Why or why not?

3. How does a relationship affect us?

4. What are some of the results of a healthy and unhealthy relationship?
   a. Healthy

      i.

      ii.

b. Unhealthy

   i.

   ii.

5. What are the some of the negative effects of stress?

Glossary

Glossary of Terms (1, 2, 3, 4, 5, 6, 7, 8, 9, 10, 11, 12, 13)

Abrasion: This is a superficial wound caused by a scrapping of the skin due to friction, grinding, and or rubbing.

Abuse: This is the systematic negative behavior in a relationship to gain and or maintain power/control over another. The directed behavior is expressed through mistreatment, cruelty, violence, intimidation, and or other negatively based reinforcers that are regularly repeated to achieve sustain control over another.

Acculturation: The process of the cultural modification of an individual or group, through adapting or borrowing beliefs and behaviors from another culture as a result of prolonged contact. Acculturation can be reciprocal and is apparent by changes in common attitudes, values, preferences, language, and beliefs.

Airborne Transmission: This is the mechanism in how an aerosol pathogen is spread. Usually in this form, its portal of entry into a susceptible host is through the lungs. The portal of exit is through the small respiratory droplets that have become aerosolized where the pathogen may travel on dust particles and or droplets from a cough, exhale, huff, laugh, or sneeze. These pathogens are loaded with infected particles and can travel over greater distances by air currents or liger in the air similar to imperceptible vapors.

Allergies: This is a hypersensitivity that evokes an immune system response to a regularly harmless substance. The reaction may vary from discomfort to a severe reaction up to and including death of the allergic subject. Again, the degree of the reaction may vary dependent on the susceptibility and tolerance ability of the client.

Angina: Is a type of chest pain caused by the reduction of blood flow to the heart muscle. The pain is primarily denoted in the chest, spreading to the shoulders, arms, and neck of the thoracic outlet area. Angina is classically described as: squeezing, pressure, heaviness, tightness, or pain in the chest; the condition is also called angina pectoris.

---

[1] http://www.cdc.gov/

[2] http://www.nimh.nih.gov

[3] http://www.merriam-webster.com/dictionary/

[4] http://www.medterms.com

[5] http://www.oxforddictionaries.com

[6] http://health.utah.gov/epi/diseases

[7] http://www.rightdiagnosis.com

[8] http://www.who.int/en/

[9] http://www.news-medical.net

[10] Jordan, R. (2013). *Basic Client Care: Client and Personal Care* [PowerPoint presentation and Lecture, Fall, 2013].

[11] Jordan, R. (2013). *Basic Client Care: Client Assessment* [PowerPoint presentation and Lecture, Fall, 2013].

[12] Jordan, R. (2013). *Basic Client Care: Support Equipment* [PowerPoint presentation and Lecture, Fall, 2013].

[13] Jordan, R. (2013). *Basic Client Care: Professional Communications* [PowerPoint presentation and Lecture, Fall, 2013].

Apical Pulse: The rhythmical throbbing by the regular contractions of the heart heard from over the apex of the heart or when palpated or detected.

Asepsis: The absence or state of being free of pathogenic microorganisms. This process is to decrease or remove pathogens that produce sepsis or septic disease.

Asthma: A respiratory condition that causes difficulty breathing through spasms and constriction of the bronchial airways.

Baseline Vitals: These first set of vital measurements represent a background level or an initial statistical measurement of an individual's physiological status. They are comparatively measured and documented to monitor, detect, determine, and calculate possible changes in the subject's condition.

Bedpan: This shallow receptacle is utilized by a bedridden client for waste elimination; it can be made of plastic or metal.

Brachial: The area from the shoulder to the elbow of an arm or forelimb of a person.

Bradycardia: This is a slower than normal heart rate. An average heart rate is considered 60-100 BPM at rest. When the rate is below this average, the results may be symptoms of fatigue, weakness, dizziness, and or fainting in a client with bradycardia.

Bias: Is the prejudice in favor of a group, person, or thing when compared with something similar. This favorable consideration can be considered unfair.

Bloodborne Pathogen: A pathogenic agent of disease spread from one person to another through contact with blood or other OPIM.

Blood Glucose Level: This is also known as blood sugar level; this reading is the indication of the amount of sugar in the bloodstream. The levels of blood sugar become significant when considering if a person is developing or has developed diabetes. Low or high blood sugar levels may significantly impact the type and course of care.

Blood Pressure: This is the measurable pressure of the circulating blood against the walls of the blood vessels.

Bronchitis: An inflammatory condition that involves the air passages leading and into the lungs; structures involved include: the trachea, main stem bronchus, bronchi, and bronchioles.

Carotid Pulse: The rhythmical throbbing by the regular contractions of the heart felt over the carotid artery, which lies between the larynx and the sternocleidomastoid muscle in the neck, used to assess CPR effectiveness.

Cardiac Catheterization (angioplasty): This is a medical procedure that involves passing a thin flexible tube (catheter) into either the right or left side of the heart. The procedure is used to diagnose and treat some heart conditions. Common points of access utilized in the procedure are the groin or the arm.

Catheter: A hollow tubular flexible medical device used primarily to pass fluid, through injection or withdraw, as well as to distend passageways; common places of insertion are blood vessels, the heart, bladder, canals, passageways, or body cavities.

Cerebrovascular Accident (CVA): This is also called a Stroke; an abnormal condition of the brain characterized by occlusion by an embolus, thrombus, or cerebrovascular hemorrhage or vasospasm, resulting in ischemia (swelling) of the brain tissues normally perfused by the damaged vessels. When a stroke occurs, the blood supply to the brain is restricted or blocked; the resulting interruption or loss results in deprivation of oxygen and nutrients to the brain tissues. The victim may suffer paralysis, speech defect, aphasia, sensory change, confusion, weakness, and even death. A stroke is a medical emergency and prompt treatment is crucial to minimize damage, residual effects, and or complication.

Chain of Infection: A model of the sequential infection process that begins with a Pathogen/Infectious Agent, Source/Reservoir, Portal of Exit (from the reservoir), Mode of Transmission, and Portal of Entry into a Susceptible Host. By understanding the characteristics of each link in the chain, healthcare practitioners may provide support in protecting vulnerable clients and aid in breaking the chain of infection.

Chest Tube: This specialized catheter is inserted through the rib space into the thoracic pleural space to remove air and/or fluid from the surrounding lung cavity. This aids in restoring negative pressure in the pleural space allowing the lungs to fully expand and return to normal function. They are commonly used when a lung has been collapsed due to traumatic injury, chest surgical procedures, and or spontaneous events. The chest tube may be either attached to a drainage device and or a water seal chest drainage device.

Cold: Also called the common cold, this illness is a contagious upper respiratory system viral infection that includes the nose, throat, sinuses, eustachian tubes, trachea, larynx, bronchial tubes, and lung fields.

Communication: A process by which information is exchanged between individuals through a common system of symbols, signs, and or behavior. Communications are considered information—written or oral, disclosed or transmitted directly or indirectly—including information revealed through observation.

Communication Pitfalls: Personal behaviors, habits, differences, or a drawback that can hinder and or negate open communication.

Community-Acquired Infection: An infection contracted in the social or community setting, primarily the term is used to distinguish from a nosocomial, or hospital-acquired infection or disease.

Condition: A state of health that may be acute, chronic, temporary, or permanent that indicates the occurrence of an injury, disorder, or illness. Conditions may restrict, limit, modify, or change the regular state and or existing functionality of a person.

Contusion: A bruising or injury to the skin from a blunt blow or crushing, the damage usually does not break the skin though it still ruptures the small blood vessels.

Convulsions: This condition is an uncontrollable violent shaking of the body due to uncontrolled, involuntary muscle contractions. Some neurological conditions may precipitate abnormal electrical activity in the brain with the resulting physical manifestations being convulsions, sensory disturbances, and or loss of consciousness.

Cultural Assimilation: A process where individual and or group culture is integrated in to the larger or more dominant group's culture. The incorporated group's culture undergoes a change in which their traditions, beliefs, and language become absorbed and nearly indistinguishable from the dominant established cultural beliefs, traditions, and language.

Cultural Diversity: The variety of human cultures and mixtures of individuals and groups of varied backgrounds, experiences, styles, perceptions, values, and beliefs. Traditions play a large part in developing diversity among cultures.

Cyanosis: This is the bluish, grayish, or dark purple discoloration of the mucous membrane, skin, lips, nail bed, fingertips, and or toe tips due to insufficient oxygen.

Death: The end of life of a person or organism, a permanent cessation of vital functions.

Dehydration: The process of the removal of water/moisture, sodium, and electrolytes; this may impair the body's ability to perform regular function. In severe cases, dehydration is a medical concern.

Depression: A mental illness that increases the feelings of despondency, dejection, and persistent sadness.

Diabetes: A metabolic disease and condition which affects the body's ability to produce any or enough insulin.

Diaphoresis: This is perceptible and profuse sweating.

Diastole: Heart muscle relaxation; the pressure of the arteries when the heart is at rest.

Direct Contact Transmission: The immediate transmission of a pathogen to a susceptible host through direct contact: skin, mouth, open wound, touching, biting, kissing and sexual contact considered person to person contact.

Discrimination: The practice of unfairly or unequal treatment a person or group of people differently from other people or groups of people. Discrimination can occur whenever a difference is perceived and acted on with the intent of establishing privileges or prohibitions on particular individual(s) based on the perceived differences. Discrimination has been based on a variety of standards including; employment, housing, education, race, age, sex, nationality, disability, and religion.

Disease: An illness classification that affects an animal, person, or plant. A disease manifests recognizable signs and symptoms that characteristically impairs regular function.

Disinfection: A process that eliminates many or all pathogenic microorganisms on inanimate objects.

Documentation: The process in which materials that provide official information or evidence serve as an official record; the record usually contains substantial information, i.e. personal, procedural, diagnosis, treatment plan, medical history, etc.

Domestic Violence: Abusive behavior used by persons in a relationship in relation to establishing control over one partner in the relationship.

Drain Tube: A device inserted into an injury, surgical site, and or wound to remove an over accumulation of blood, pus, or other unwanted fluid and materials that may hinder the injury from recovery.

Droplet Transmission: This is the transmission mechanism in how droplet infectious agents are spread through the air. Contagious droplets produced by an infected host are propelled a short distance through: coughing, talking, huffing, laughing, sneezing, or through strong exhalation. The usual portals of entry for the droplet pathogens are: eyes, nose, mouth, or other areas with exposed mucosal linings. These pathogen loaded droplets are large—generally greater than 10 micrometers and are unable to stay suspended in the air. Droplets can generally travel short distances from 3 to 6 feet from the host and are generally unaffected by specialized air handling or standard control of room pressures. It is greatly suspected that large droplet transmission is the primary method for nosocomial infection transmission.

Dyspnea: This condition is the uncomfortable awareness of having the urge to breathe, a difficulty with breathing, or shortness of breath; it is caused or aggravated by lack of oxygenation of the bloodstream.

Edema: The excessive accumulation of fluids in the soft tissues resulting in swelling due to an abnormally increased volume of serous fluid.

Emesis Basin: This kidney shaped shallow basin is used to collect client's vomit, bile, excessive salivation, spittle, sputum, and various orally expressed fluids. Primarily used for relief of the bed ridden or for client's with restricted movement.

Elements of Communication: Essential components of communication comprised of Sender, Receiver, or Message; by eliminating any one of these essential components there can be no communication.

Eye and Face Protection: These are a type of personal protective equipment made from see-through materials that reduce or prevent the risk of airborne, droplet, and contact transmission pathogens from blood and body fluid of any patient. They are standard facial precautions for all healthcare workers.

Febrile/Fever: A characterization of an elevated body temperature, usually due to an introduced pathogen. Generally, the condition requirements for being considered febrile are that the subject's body temperature is above 100° F (37.8° C). Additional symptoms may include feeling cold or chilled even though the subject has an elevated body temperature.

Feeding Tube: This is a flexible tube used to provide nutrition to patients who cannot obtain nutrition through swallowing.

Femoral Pulse: The rhythmical throbbing by the regular contractions located where the femoral artery passes through the groin.

Fomite Transmission: The mechanism of transmission through an inanimate object that is capable of transmitting an infectious pathogen. The inanimate object (brush, chair, clothing, dish, doorknob, book, desk, phone, etc.) that has become contaminated through contact with an infectious agent or organism then serves as a means of contact transmission from infected host to susceptible host.

Fowler's: An inclined sitting up position with the knees slightly bent for comfort and support. The inclined sitting position can vary from 15 degrees to 90 degrees. The Fowler's position is used to promote oxygenation and relief of respiratory distress by alleviating compression of the chest due to gravity and the promotion of the collection of intra-abdominal fluids in the lower part of abdomen.

Fracture: A disruption or break in the continuity of the boney tissues and or cartilaginous structures.

Gait Belt: A transfer device used to safely relocate clients from one position or location to another. By placing the gait belt around a client's waist and assisting their ambulatory transfer, the healthcare practitioner may more safely convey clients that have problems with balance and movement stability. The belt is generally made from a cotton material with a sturdy and durable buckle.

Generalization: This is a broad statement or belief based on a limited number of facts, incomplete data, and or assessments; for example, the beliefs, values behaviors, etc., of a group of persons or situation.

Hand Protection: These are fitted coverings for the hands of the healthcare provider. The gloves are disposable and composed usually of latex or vinyl to provide protection to the healthcare professional from blood, urine, saliva, drainage, wound seepage, lesions, open wounds, and other potentially infectious materials during contact periods of client management. In addition, these personal protective equipment coverings also reduce the risk for clients who require a reverse isolation environment. Through wearing hand protection, the healthcare provider reduces the risk of contamination and transmitting pathogens while maintaining a safe and clean environment for client treatment. Hand protection can be provided for the healthcare practitioner for clean and or sterile environment treatment options.

Hand Washing: Washing hands with soap and water is the best way to reduce the number of germs on them and is considered the foremost way to fight the spread of disease or illness. If soap and water are not available, use an alcohol-based hand sanitizer that contains at least 60% alcohol.

Headache: This is simply, pain in the head.

Health: The condition of the mind, body, and or emotions, moreover the degree to which their state of being is free from illness or injury.

Heart Rate: The timed number of heartbeats (contractions) usually measured in a minute. The measure of cardiac activity can aid in determining the condition and general health of the individual. The pulse is often utilized to estimate the heart rate.

Hypertension: This is a condition where the pressure of the blood flowing through the arteries of the body is higher than it should be regularly; with this condition, the blood pressure is persistently elevated above the normal region. The ranges of blood pressure are considered the following: Normal: Systolic is below 120 mm Hg and Diastolic is less than 80 mm Hg; Prehypertension: Systolic range is 120–139 mm Hg and the Diastolic range is 80–89 mm Hg; Hypertension Stage 1: Systolic range is 140–159 mm Hg and the Diastolic range is 90–99 mm Hg; Hypertension Stage 2: Systolic range is 160 mm Hg or higher and the Diastolic range 100 mm Hg or higher.

Hypothermia: A characterization of a decreased body temperature when body temperature falls below 95°F (35°C). Hypothermia is a medical emergency and a potentially fatal condition when the body's internal mechanisms are unable to retain the heat being lost due to a drop in core temperature. This most often occurs in a body when it is exposure to cold weather or immersion in cold water for a period of time. The characteristic symptoms that occur are, shivering and mental confusion as the body's temperature drops.

Ideal Communications: Ideal Communications is the concept of providing the best circumstances in which shared information can be provided and received by the participants of the communication.

Infection: An invasion or compromise of tissues with the multiplication of an invading pathogenic organism.

Infectious Agent: An organism capable of producing infection able to live in or on the tissue of a living animal; may not necessarily cause disease. In a susceptible host, the infectious agent can create a cycle of: cellular failure, tissue failure, organ failure, and finally system failure due to competitive metabolism, toxins, and intracellular replication.

Influenza: This is an acute highly infectious respiratory and intestinal viral disease, commonly known as flu.

Labored Breathing: This is an abnormal state of respiration for the client, it is characterized by an increased effort to breathe; the efforts may include the use of accessory muscles of respiration, stridor, grunting, or nasal flaring.

Laceration: A deep, cut, tear, split, or gash in the skin as a result of an injury.

Lateral: This refers to a client position of lying on their side or being viewed from a side (a lateral view).

Listening Factors: An activity that involves four essential elements represented in Perception, Interpretation, Evaluation, and Action. A healthcare practitioner primarily uses these factors in providing quality care when attentively listening in a conversation to improve their ability to comprehend and respond to a client's message.

Lithotomy: This refers to a client position of lying on the back with the legs spread apart, thighs acutely flexed towards the abdomen, and legs may be assisted in this position by the use of stirrups to support the feet and legs.

Mask: A piece of medical equipment or device worn over the nose and mouth closely through which supplemental oxygen is supplied from a reservoir or additional source to aid in respiratory support. This supportive equipment may be augmented to enhance oxygen supplementation by attaching an oxygen reservoir bag creating a semi closed breathing circuit.

Medical Record: This document is a case history of chronological written accounts of a patient's medical history, complaints, examinations, physician's physical findings, results of diagnostic tests, therapeutic procedures, treatments, medications, and resulting effects.

Message: The symbols in a communication that represent the idea. This may be a verbal message or a nonverbal message done via face-to-face or another form of transmission.

Microorganisms: These are single celled organisms that can only be seen with a microscope.

Myocardial Infarction (Heart Attack): A heart attack is a result of interrupted blood flow to the heart, which can damage or destroy the heart muscle. When the blood flow to a part of the heart is blocked for a long enough period time, the part of the heart muscle that is deprived becomes damaged or dies. Usually this occurs when an occlusion, blood clot, or severe stenosis blocks the flow of blood through a coronary artery.

Nasal Cannula: An oxygen delivering device of a flexible light weight plastic tubing used to deliver supplemental oxygen or airflow to a client. In design, the tube splits into a loop which fits over the client's ears, the loop has dual prongs that are slightly curved and are placed in the nostrils of the client. The extended end length of the tube has a fitted end that is attached to supplemental oxygen tank or wall regulator.

Nausea: An uneasiness or queasiness of the stomach; also an urge to vomit.

NG, NJ, ND, and PEG Tubes: The insertion point of the feeding tube is indicated in the abbreviation (NG) nasogastric, insertion place is through the (N) Nasal; with the tube end placement indicated in the last letter of the abbreviation (G) gastric. An (NJ) nasojejunal, (N) Nasal, (J) Jejunum ND The NG, NJ, and ND tubes are placed to provide nutrition and supplemental aid to patients who are unable to acquire adequate oral nutrition. (PEG) tube stands for Percutaneous Endoscopic Gastric Tube; which is a feeding tube which punctures through the external abdominal wall through to the stomach. This is done with the guidance of an endoscopic procedure for the tube placement. The PEG tube is a means of providing nutrition to patients who are unable to acquire adequate oral nutrition due to trauma, injury, paralysis, or other conditions that may prohibit regular means of oral nutrition.

Nonverbal: This is the part or portion of communication not involving or using words, speech, or vocals when communicating. It may include body language, para-linguistics, posture, haptics, gestures, facial expressions, and or the use of the environment. The nonverbal message generated by the source may carry considerable content. In most communications the nonverbal message is used best to express or emphasize complex emotional, situational, intense, and or the degree of importance of information to the receiver. This portion of communication can be both intentional and unintentional.

Nosocomial Infection: A localized or systemic infection transmitted as a result of treatment in either a hospital or a healthcare facility.

Obesity: This is the condition characterized by gaining excessive weight and retaining the overweight condition.

Other Potentially Infectious Materials (OPIM): These are human bodily fluids that can potentially be infectious or contaminated, and could be a vehicle of transmission for pathogens. The following is a list of some potential materials: amniotic fluid, semen, vaginal secretions, cerebrospinal fluid, synovial fluid, pleural fluid, pericardial fluid, peritoneal fluid, saliva, any other body fluid that are visibly contaminated with blood such as saliva or vomitus, and all body fluids.

Orthopnea: This condition of discomfort and or difficulty in breathing occurs when lying down and may be relieved upon changing the client's position to upright sitting or standing position.

Oxemitry: This is the determination of the level of oxygen saturation of circulating arterial blood using an oximeter.

Oxygen Saturation: This is the state of having an amount of dissolved oxygen bound to hemoglobin in the blood in the client's bloodstream. The value of saturation indicated is usually expressed as a percentage; normal saturation levels are considered 95%-100%.

Patient Positioning: A method of deliberate placement, arraignment, or designation of the patient's body, posture, or structures of the body to promote and or facilitate an examination, surgery, therapeutic, physiologic and or psychological well-being. An example of common patient positions are the following: Fowler's, Lateral, Lithotomy, Prone, Recumbent, Sims, and Trendelenberg.

Personal Protective Equipment (PPE): These healthcare tools are a part of standard precautions for all healthcare workers. Properly emplaced these safe guards assist in the prevention of exposure to contagious and or pathogenic agents; through reducing incidental exposure to the client's and practitioner's skin, mucous membrane, possible compromised immune systems, integumentary conditions, and or illnesses from contact with blood and body fluid of each other. PPE includes protective laboratory clothing, disposable gloves, eye protection, and face masks.

Physiologic Need: These biological qualities are essential in the normal function of living organisms. The restriction, deprivation, or removal of any one of these needs or collective benefits of these can cause severe repercussions in varying degrees up to and including the cessation/death of the organism. The basic/physiologic needs include the following: air, food, drink, sleep/rest, shelter/protection from harmful elements, and waste elimination.

Portal of Entry: The access point of where a pathogen gains access or entry into a susceptible host. Portals of entry may vary consider the following examples; catheters, mucous membrane, possible compromised immune systems, compromised integumentary conditions, cuts, lesions, injection sites, and or natural body orifices.

Portal of Exit: Considers the medium and the mode of transmission the pathogen leaves the reservoir; cough, sneeze, through blood, feces, mucus, or saliva.

Post-Traumatic Stress Disorder (PTSD): This is a mental health condition brought on by an excessively disturbing event that impacts the participant or observer.

Prejudice: An adverse irrational judgment or opinion formed beforehand or without knowledge or examination of the facts directed against an individual or group solely based on their supposed characteristics.

Privileged Information: Sensitive information protected by law in relation to healthcare settings intended for specific or designated authorized individuals, organizations, and or purposes.

Prone: A client position that is indicated by the patient lying face down with arms bent comfortably at the elbow and padded with the arm boards positioned forward. This position is also indicated by the client lying on their ventral surface or called a recumbent face down position.

Proximity: This is the state, quality, or sense indicating the nearness in space, time, or relationship. Proximity is always relative in fact of being near, close, or next to another subject.

Pulse: This is the rhythmic throbbing of the arterial flow from the contractions of the heart, usually measured in beats per minute.

Receiver: The person or group to whom the message is directed in a communication. The receiver can be an individual, team, department, unit, organization, and or a populace en masse.

Recumbent: This position denotes that the subject is lying down or reclining, specifically in a position of comfort or rest.

Reservoir: Considered in the chain of infection is the link of continual source of infection of an infected host; this can be the blood, saliva, sores, bodily fluid, or other potentially infectious materials.

Respectful Communications: In Respectful Communication with clients, the healthcare practitioner demonstrates consideration, understanding, and or appropriate regard for someone due to their value, achievements, importance, admirable qualities, or position—when having a conversation or communicating with them.

Respirator (PPE): A device that is designed to remove harmful contaminates, dusts, fumes, and or vapors from inhalation. There are two primary categories of respirators: an air-purifying respirator, a device which forces contaminated air through a filtering element to reduce or remove harmful contaminates, and the airline respirator, in which an alternate compressed supply of fresh air is delivered through to a self-contained breathing apparatus. Both classifications of respirators apply different techniques to reduce or remove the airborne hazard.

Respiration: The act of inhaling and exhaling air for oxygen and gas exchange.

Respiratory Distress: A condition described as difficulty or distress with breathing, which can be the result of disease, illness, or psychological experience; even with no physiological basis. The condition can affect the ability to exchange oxygen for patients with lung disease.

Restraints: These are any manual method, physical device, or equipment applied which limits or restricts a client's movement or freedom. The use of unwilling confinement, control, or restraints on a client may only be utilized if the client is a danger or threat to themselves or others. A physicians consent and order must be obtained in order to apply restraints. Physical or chemical restraints must never be used on a client for the convenience of staff.

Seizure: This condition is abnormal electrical in the brain with the physical manifestations of convulsions, sensory disturbances, and or loss of consciousness.

Sender: The person or group with the information and the reason for communicating. This can be an individual, team, department, unit, organization, and or a populace en masse.

Sexually Transmitted Infections (STI/STD): A various number of diseases that are primarily contracted through sexual intercourse and or other intimate sexual contact.

Shallow Breathing: an abnormal respiration pattern indicated by slow, shallow, and generally producing ineffective inspirations and expirations with low tidal volumes.

Signs: These are objective measurable indications of complaint, disease, illness, or injury; especially as observed and interpreted by a healthcare professional providing evidence of the existence of the client's complaint, disease, illness, or injury.

Sims: A position in which the patient lies on one side with the side down leg/thigh slightly flexed and the opposite leg/thigh acutely flexed up towards the abdomen; the arm of the side that is down is marginally behind (not under) the body for client comfort, and the opposite arm is positioned in flexed and in front according to the patient's comfort. The head, forward arm, and leg may be supported with pillows or cushions for patient comfort. The Sims position is used to facilitate examinations and for clients whom have difficulty lying in a recumbent position due to injury, illness, or contraindicated conditions.

Skeletal Traction: This is a method of drawing, pulling, or extending through a pin or wire surgically inserted into an affected bone to immobilize, position, and or align a fractured bone or structure properly during and to facilitate the healing process.

Skin Traction: This method of drawing, pulling, or extending through a mechanism consisting of adhesive or nonadhesive strapping attached to the skin surrounding the structure or limb to immobilize, position, and or align a structure properly during and to facilitate the healing process.

S.O.A.P. Notes: These are a uniform note format to document, organize, and chart patient progression; SOAP notes are primarily employed by health care providers, auditors, and accreditation councils to easily review client records.

Sprain: A wrenching, twisting, stretching, or tearing motion resulting in damage or injury to the tendon, or fibrous connective tissues involved.

Stereotyping: This is regarding a conventional, formulaic, and oversimplified conception, opinion, or image that embodies a set image or type of person or thing for classification.

Sterilization: Describes a process that destroys or eliminates all forms of microbial life and is carried out by physical or chemical methods.

Sterile Technique: This technique is in reference to an aseptic procedure performed under sterile conditions. Primarily utilized in hospitals or healthcare setting for procedures performed under specific conditions to minimize and reduce contamination and possible pathogenic exposure.

Strain: A wrenching, twisting, stretching, or tearing motion resulting in damage or injury done to the muscular tissues involved.

Stress: The body's response to internal, unresolved conflict/forces.

Stroke: This is a sudden blockage, interruption, or rupture of a blood vessel that results in the sudden death of brain cells due to lack of oxygen.

Suctioning: This is regarded as the act or process of removing secretions or fluids through the use of negative pressure by means of a tube and a device (suction pump/suction bulb) that operates on negative pressure. The suctioning procedure is primarily used for clients that unable to clear or remove the secretions or debris on their own from the site. Care and special skills may be required for cleanliness, care, treatment, and or respiratory therapies.

Supine: A position with the patient lying down on their back or dorsal side down and face up, predominantly with arms comfortably at their sides.

Support Equipment: These can be mechanical devices, items, and or tools which aid the healthcare practitioner in providing protection, care, security, comfort, and or services to clients during their procedures, treatment, and or care.

Surgical Mask: A specially designed procedural mask that is intended to eliminate or reduce the spread of infectious contaminants. They are worn during surgery and various procedures by healthcare practitioners to catch droplet and aerosols from the wearer's mouth and nose.

Susceptible Host: This is an organism that can be infected or likely to be affected by pathogens which could cause a disease, infection, or condition.

Symptom: These are subjective sensations that are not quantifiable or cannot be measured. Though they are difficult to ascertain or quantify they can be important in determining a medical prognosis as well as treatment plans.

Systole: Heart muscle contraction; the force required to pump the blood out of the heart into the aorta and the arteries to cause circulation.

Tachycardia: This is a faster than normal heart rate. An average heart rate is considered 60-100 BPM at rest. When the rate is above the average (typically 100 beats per minute or higher) the results may be symptoms of fatigue, faintness, shortness of breath, and or feeling that the heart is thumping in a client with tachycardia.

Tachypnea: This condition is defined as having an abnormally rapid respiration rate, usually a respiration rate over 20 breaths per minute.

Temperature: Is considered the level of heat in the body of a living organism, usually about 98.6 degrees.

Traction: This is the utilization of pulling tension to treat muscle and skeleton disorders; by facilitating immobilization, specific positions, and or alignment of body structures properly this treatment method is used to facilitate the healing process.

Trauma: A deeply disturbing event or serious injury to an individual from an incident involving violence or an accident producing shock to the body.

Trendelenburg: This is a supine position described as the patient is placed on a table or bed with the feet inclined higher than their head upper section to approximately 45 degrees so that the head is lower than the rest of the body. Support is required to keep the patient from slipping from the table.

Tubes: A flexible hollow cylinder particularly used to facilitate the passage of fluids through removal or deposit.

Urinal: This is a portable plastic or other receptacle primarily used by bed ridden or fall risk male patients to urinate in they are not ambulatory.

Vaccination: This is a method of prepared treatment to prevent the spread of viral, bacterial, and or disease causing agents to assist in the development of the treated subject's immune system.

Vector Transmission: This is an indirect transmission of an infectious agent that may occur when an infected insect, animal, or arachnid vector bites or touches a susceptible host. The most common vectors are blood sucking insects such as mosquitoes, fleas, lice, biting flies and bugs which may transmit an infectious agent through feeding.

Verbal: This is the part or portion of communication involving or use of words, speech, or vocals when communicating. Included in the vocal communication are enunciation, stress, tone, inflection, rhythm, and sounds that may convey additional content. Written language is also considered a portion of verbal communication.

Vital Signs: are the statistical measurements of an individual's physiological status. They are comparatively measured and documented to monitor, detect, determine, and calculate possible changes in the subject's condition.

Vomiting: This is the voluntary or involuntary evacuation of the contents of the of stomach contents through the oropharynx and or nasopharynx passageway(s) also known as throwing up.

Answers

Chapter 1: Communication

1. The three components of communication are sender, message, and receiver.

2. Encoding occurs when the message sender puts the information into a form that the receiver can understand.

3. a. The patient may eat only two meals a day, and therefore, will take only two pills.

   b. The nurse should tell the patient to take one pill three times a day with food. The pills should be taken about 4–6 hours apart.

4. About 55 percent of our message is transmitted through body language. Body language includes facial expressions, eye contact, body position, stance, and/or motion.

5. When entering the room, tell the patient who you are and what you plan to do. Keeping the patient aware of what is happening helps to keep the patient comfortable and agreeable to the procedures that you must perform.

6. Cellphones can be used in hospitals much like they are used in daily life. However, you must keep confidentiality in mind when discussing a patient. Information shared on a cellphone is not confidential and may be overheard by someone.

7. The patient's culture may determine that withdrawing blood is unacceptable and that belief would make the test unacceptable to him. Possibly explaining the reason for the blood test would help him be more amenable to it, but he may not ever come to terms with having blood drawn.

8. Knowing how another person may be sending or perceiving information helps with understanding the message or delivering information to another person.

Chapter 2: Vital Signs

1. Age, pain, disease, gender, activity, obesity, emotions, heredity, stimulants, medications.

2. The patient may have a wrist injury

3. Diastolic

4. 100–160

5. Identify yourself and identify the patient

6. Carotid, brachial, radial, temporal, apical, femoral, popliteal, dorsalis pedis, posterior tibial

7. Tell him or her that you're checking their respirations, as just knowing that will change the rate.

8. Difficulty breathing in other than an upright position

9. The patient may be in critical condition

10. Fever

Chapter 3: Infection Control

1. *Normal flora* are the microorganisms that naturally occur within the human body.

2. *Protozoans* are single-celled organisms that can invade a human and cause disease. Three types produce disease in humans: amoeba, flagellates, and sporozoans. *Entamoeba histolytica* is an amoeba that lives in the human intestinal tract without problem. However, if it invades the colon's mucous membrane, it can cause amoebic dysentery. *Giardia lamblia* is the flagellate that causes giardiasis, a type of diarrhea. This flagellate attaches itself to the surface of the small intestine and can become so prevalent that it interferes with nutrient absorption. Malaria is spread by mosquitoes carrying the sporozoa *Plasmodium*. *Plasmodium* multiplies in the liver and then invades the red blood cells, destroying them so extensively as to cause severe anemia.

3. A *nosocomial infection* is one that is picked up in a hospital; *community-acquired infections* are picked up through contact with people, animals, foods, water, etc., that are common in our environment.

4. *Fomite bacterial transmission* is bacterium is on a nonliving object, such as bedding, towels, and locker rooms, from which they move to a patient. The fungus *Trichophyton*—the source of athletes' foot—is transmitted from locker room floors.

5. The six steps in the chain of infection: (1) infectious agent, (2) reservoir, (3) portal of exit, (4) mode of transmission, (5) portal of entry, and (6) susceptible host. If one of these steps is missing, the infection will not occur.

6. Handwashing is the easiest way to break the chain of infection. Follow these steps to correctly wash your hands:

    1. Wet your hands with running water.

    2. Apply enough soap to cover the hands. Regular soap is as effective as antibacterial soap.

    3. Lather well.

4. Rub the hands together, being sure to get soap to the backs of the hands, in between the fingers, under the fingernails and wrists.

5. Rinse the soap from the hands.

6. Dry hands with a single-use towel and use that towel to turn off the water.

7. *Universal precautions* are guidelines to ensure prevention of contact with blood or other potentially infectious materials such as semen, vaginal secretions, amniotic fluid, saliva in dental procedures, etc. These guidelines were developed by OSHA.

8. Personal protective equipment includes such items such as gloves, face shields or masks, eye protection, and gowns and/or lab coats. Mouthpieces, resuscitation bags, and other ventilation devices must be made available by the employer.

9. Containers to collect used needles, scalpels, broken glass, broken capillary tubes, and exposed ends of dental wires. They are made of red plastic.

10. The sequence for putting on the PPE is (1) gown, (2) mask/respirator, and eye and face protection, (3) then gloves.

Chapter 4: Patient Mobility

1. The head of the bed is elevated 30–90 degrees and the knees also elevated.

2. Because the patient has trouble breathing when lying flat.

3. (1) To prevent falls, (2) to prevent wandering, (3) to protect equipment, (4) to control agitation.

4. Follow this 10-step procedure:

    i.   Set the brake on the wheelchair so it won't move.

    ii.   Stabilize the bed so it won't move and lower it to the floor.

    iii.   Put a transfer belt around the patient's waist.

    iv.   Stand in front of the patient.

    v.   With a straight back, bend from the hips and knees and grasp the patient around the waist, holding onto the transfer belt.

    vi.   Stand erect pulling the patient up, keeping her knees between your knees.

    vii.   Pause to make sure the patient is stable.

    viii. Taking small steps, pivot the patient so her back is square with the bed.

ix.   Slowly lower patient to the bed, bending your knees and hips.

x.   Swing the patient's legs onto the bed and help her return to the recumbent position.

5. Use a patient lift.

6. For a rectal examination

7. Bedsore; pressure points; relieve pressure points with padding

8. To move a patient from one area to another; avoid injury to caregiver and patient; help in balance

Chapter 5: Special Care

1. *Physiologic needs* relate to the actual functioning of a patient's body. Healthcare workers must understand these needs to provide comfort and correct care to the patient.

2. Follow these steps:

   a. Wash your hands and put on gloves.

   b. Ask the patient to place the urinal between his legs. If the patient is unable to so, spread the patient's legs and put the urinal into place. Ask a male to put his penis in the opening at the top of the urinal. If unable to do so, assist him in positioning the penis.

   c. Position the urinal properly and hold it gently while the patient urinates.

   d. When the patient finished, carefully remove the urinal, cover it with a towel, and place it on a chair next to the bed.

   e. Assist the patient in cleaning between the legs with a damp washcloth. (If the patient is female, clean from front to back.)

   f. Dry the area between the legs.

3. An *emesis basin* catches vomitus. However, these are not used for vomiting due to their size. An *emesis bag* is used as it is larger and makes it easier to dispose of the vomitus.

4. Oral suctioning is done when a patient is unable to clear secretions from his or her mouth and throat. Nasal suctioning is done when a patient is unable to maintain a patent airway.

5. *CPR* is cardiopulmonary resuscitation. Everyone who works in the healthcare field should know CPR.

6. When patient faints, assist them to the floor. Lay the patient on the back, with legs elevated 8 to 12 inches. Loosen any clothing that may be constricting. Call for assistance from another healthcare worker to return the patient to bed when the patient has stabilized.

7. *Skeletal traction* refers to the application of pins and the use of weights and pulleys attached to the pins. Skeletal traction is frequently used for injuries to the femur, tibia, humerus, and cervical spine. Traction keeps the bones in correct alignment while healing.

8. A simple nasal mask would be used to deliver 8–10 liters per minute of oxygen.

9. Drains remove fluid that may collect around the heart following heart surgery. The drain remains in place until the flow of fluid is decreased to a minimum or has stopped.

10. Some types of tubing are nasogastric, endotracheal, gastrostomy, and chest. A nasogastric tubes is inserted through the nose and terminate in the stomach. It is used to remove the stomach contents, which includes air or fluid. An endotracheal tube is inserted via the nose but terminate in the trachea. It provides anesthesia during surgery, provides oxygen to a patient, and is used for endoscopic lung procedures. A gastrostomy tube provides nutrients to patients who cannot ingest food. The tube is inserted like a nasogastric tube or via a puncture in the abdomen that terminates in the stomach. A chest tube is inserted through the chest wall to remove air, fluids, or pus from the chest cavity. It is used to treat a pneumothorax or hemothorax.

Chapter 6: Documentation

1. The physician chart is owned by the hospital or clinic. The information in the chart is owned by the patient.

2. Medical records document patient care, ensuring that the continuity of care is appropriate.

3. Each entry should include:

   - patient name and identification number;

   - date and time;

   - observations;

   - treatment given and

   - care provider signature.

4. Electronic records are used to consolidate the paper records used previously. The conversion to electronic records is being funded by the federal government through the HITECH Act.

5. To make sure you use the correct record, look at the patient name and identification number.

6. To keep the patient information confidential, move out of the hallway. Take notes as you listen and confirm with your coworker that what you heard is correct.

7. If using a paper record, cross out the incorrect information, make the correction, and initial and date the change. If using an electronic record, create an "addendum" to the original entry, noting the correction.

8. A SOAP note is a way to format a record entry. S = Subjective; O = Objective; A = Assessment; P = Plan.

9. Military time is based on a 24-hour clock. When using military time, there is no mistaking a morning or afternoon time, as for example,1500 always means 3 hours after noon.

10. Medical records are used in legal matters. A record may be subpoenaed to provide evidence in court.

Chapter 7: Personal Health and Common Conditions

1. How does weight change our life style? Weight can change our lifestyle in several ways; most commonly known are decreased activity, energy, and lifespan. Weight gain may trigger or aggravate other secondary conditions or disease processes for example: heart disease, diabetes, arthritis, hypertension, stroke, and many others.

   a. Less activity: this is the reduction of exercise and the deterioration of capability to do exercise.

   b. Energy: through inactivity, a person's energy levels decreases as does their desire to be active.

   c. Decreased lifespan: with the onset of health conditions, an increased chance of dying from or due to a complication of a secondary condition increases.

2. Does a diet effectively work? Why or why not? We consider a diet to not effectively work alone, it has been shown that a diet with a lifestyle change increases the chances and sustains the desired effects of maintaining a targeted weight and overall health.

3. How does a relationship affect us? A relationship can affect our personal outlook, mental state, and emotional state, which effectively impacts how we negotiate our interactions with others, our desire and ability to complete tasks and the decisions that are made during the course of our daily activities.

4. What are some of the results of a healthy and unhealthy relationship?

   a. Healthy

      i. Positive outlook in resolving issues

      ii. Support structure that provides care

      iii. Reduced stress

      iv. Improved personal communication

      v. Increased healthy social activity

b. Unhealthy

    i.   Increased stress

    ii. Poor personal interaction

    ii.   Increased risk to health

    iii. Decreased immune system

    iv. Harmful relationship dynamics learned

5. What are the some of the negative effects of stress? There are many overarching negative effects of stress, some include: reduced immune system, increased risk to health, hypertension, stroke, ulcers, headaches, and even death.

Opening a Sterile Package Diagram

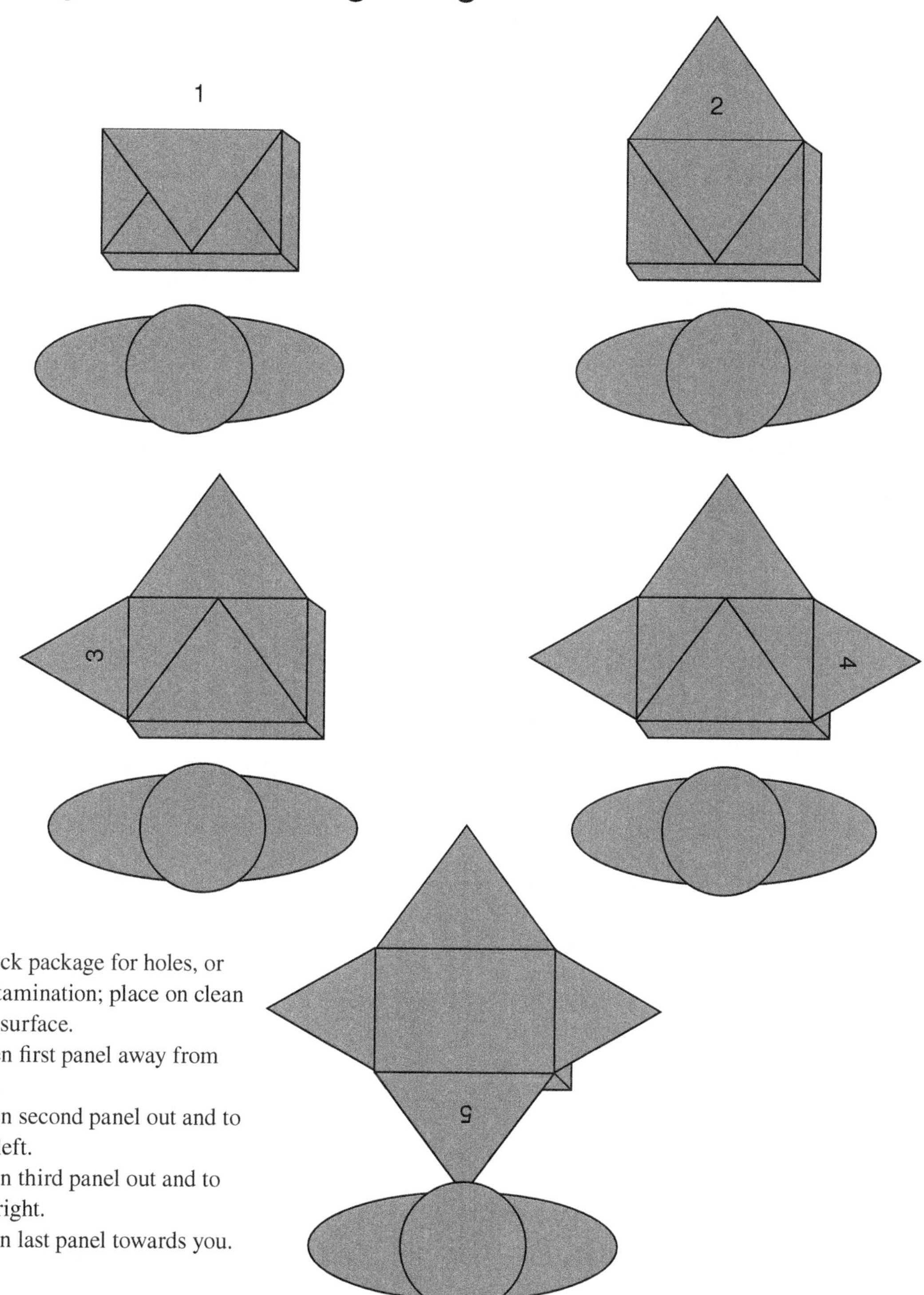

1. Check package for holes, or contamination; place on clean dry surface.
2. Open first panel away from you.
3. Open second panel out and to the left.
4. Open third panel out and to the right.
5. Open last panel towards you.

K.I.M.		
Key	**Information**	**Memory**

Name ____

BACK

FRONT

Notes: _______________________________

S

O

A

P

Name: _______________________________
Date: _______________________________
MR#: _______________________________
DOB: _______________________________
Age: _______________________________
Height: _______________________________
Allergies: _______________________________

Chief Complaint: _______________________________

Medications: _______________________________

Recent HX: _______________________________

Vitals
Heart Rate: _______________________________
BP: _______________________________
Temperature: _______________________________
Respirations: _______________________________
02 Sat: _______________________________

What Happens When???

Consider what the client goes through when they are subjected to an acute condition, illness, or tramatic event. Think of three different persons with acute conditions, illnes, or tramatic incidents. Write in the Acute Condition(s) triangle the three selected conditions. Then review and make notes in the provided and surrounding spaces as to how you figure the denoted condition effected the person's Physical, Mental, and Emotional wellbeing; what would like likely happen in the event of this condition occurring. Review them in the following order: 1. Physical; 2. Mental; 3. Emotional

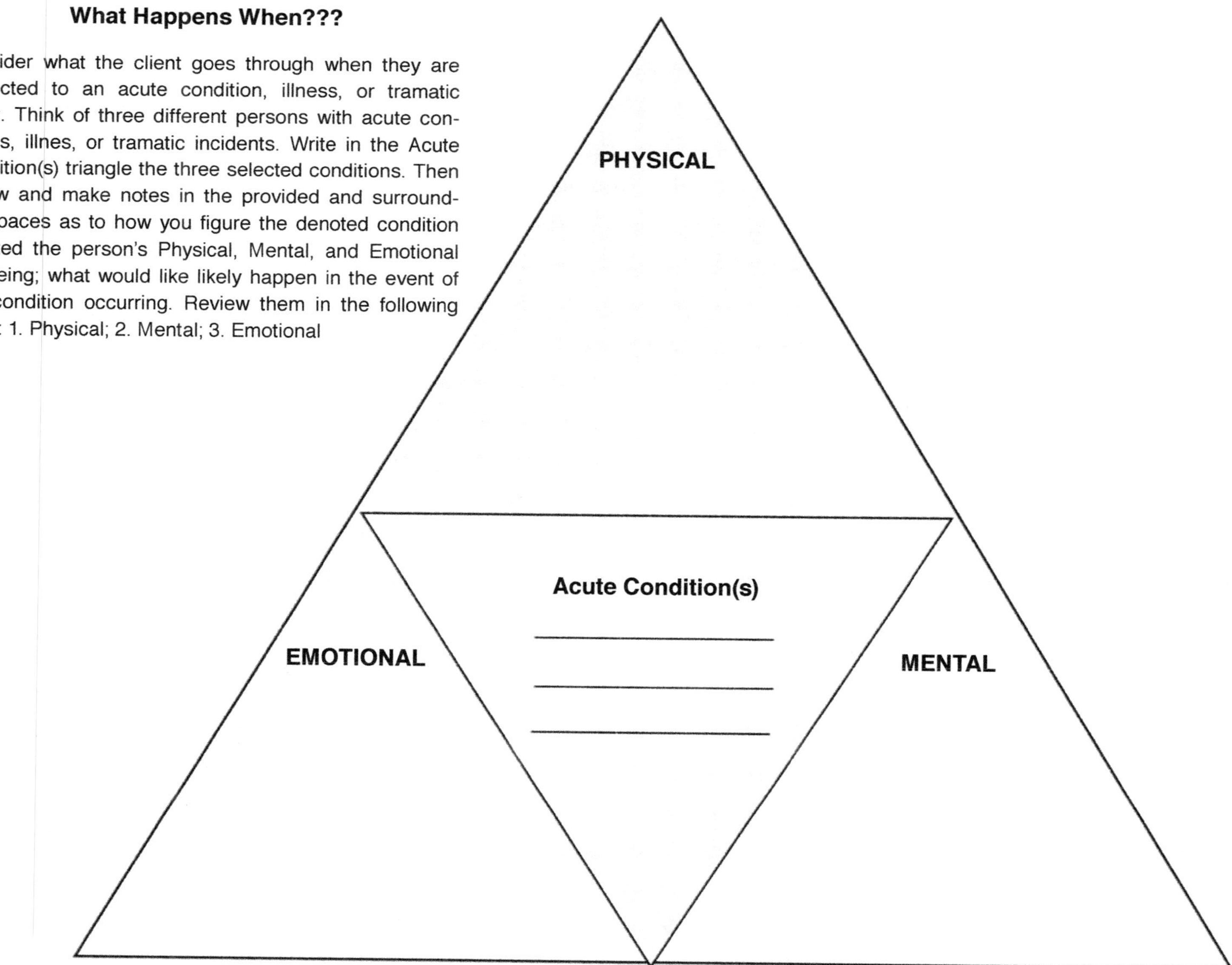

What Happens When???

Consider what the client goes through when they are subjected to a chronic condition, illness, or tramatic event. Think of three different persons with chronic conditions, illnes, or tramatic incidents. Write in the Chronic Condition(s) triangle the three selected conditions. Then review and make notes in the provided and surrounding spaces as to how you figure the denoted condition effected the person's Physical, Mental, and Emotional wellbeing; what would like likely happen in the event of this condition occurring. Review them in the following order: 1. Physical; 2. Mental; 3. Emotional

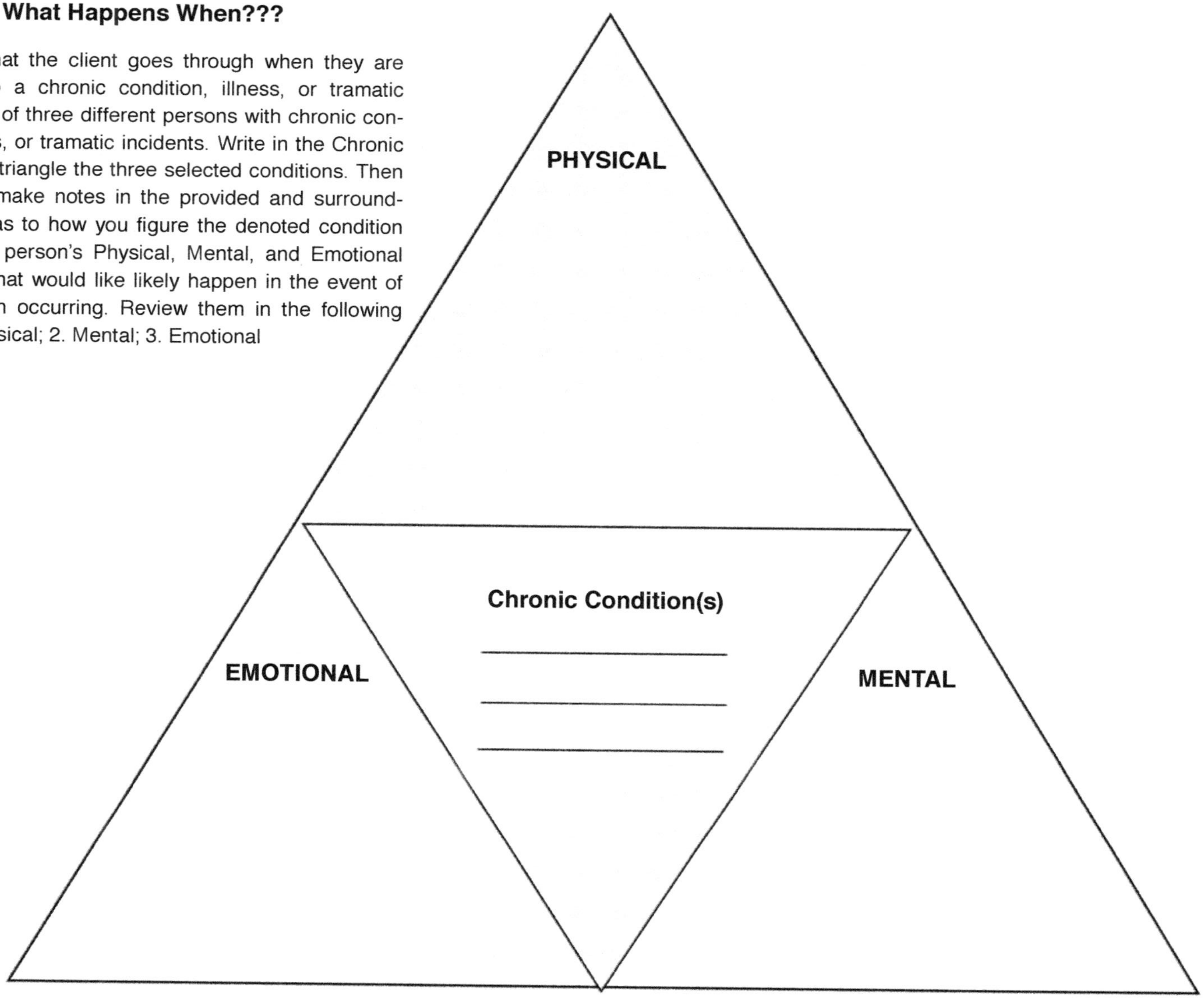

What Happens When???

Consider what happens to the vital signs of a client when a client has a condition (illness, or traumatic event). In the center triangle place a considered condition and in the additional vital areas review and make notes as to what would like likely happen in the event of this condition occurring. Review them in the following order:

1. Respiration; 2. Heart Rate; 3. Blood Pressure

What is your hypothesis why?

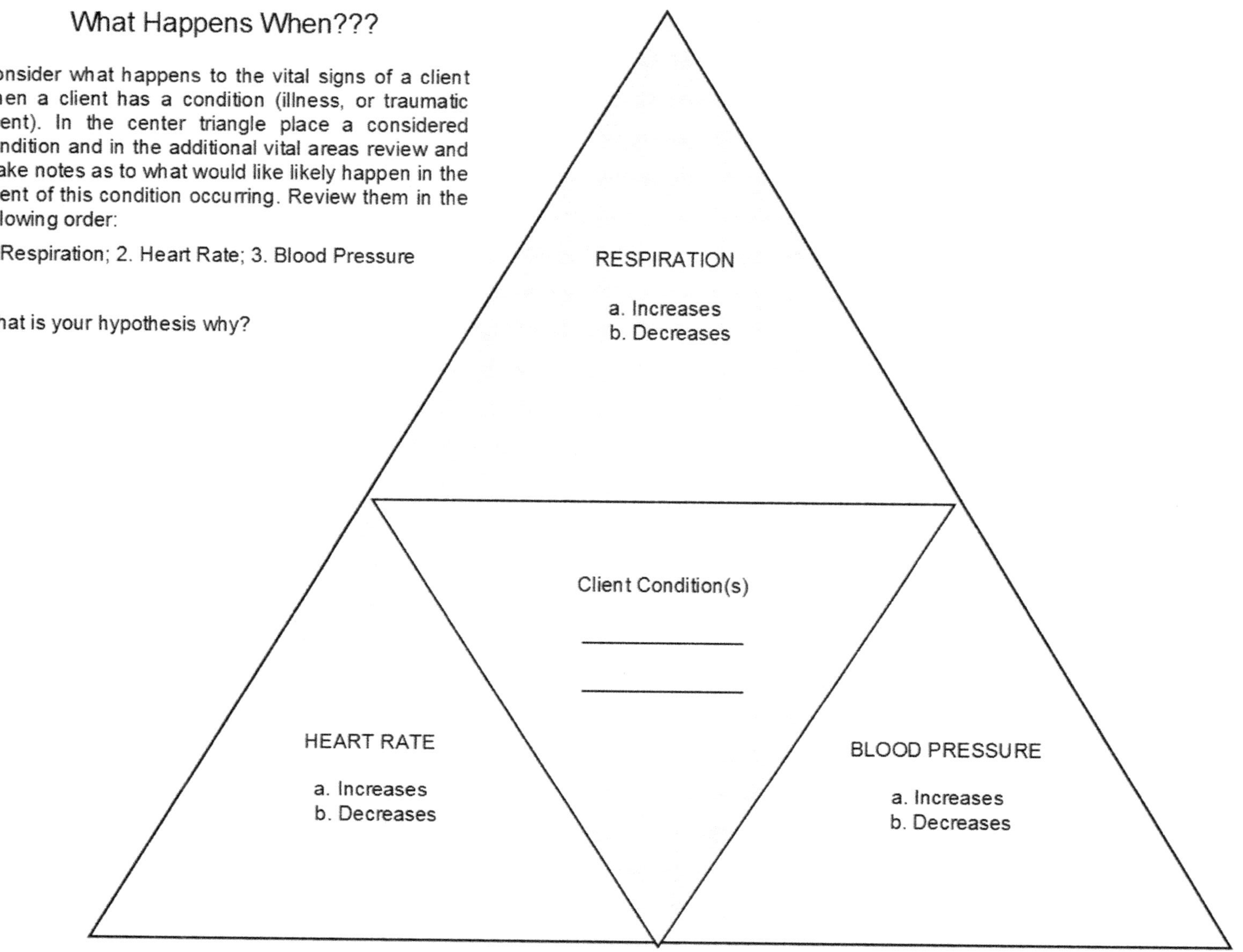

Compare or Contrast the Three

Review and or study three subjects by placing each subject in an external triangle and writing their differences or their similarities in the center triangle. Then review and make notes in the provided and surrounding spaces as to how you figure they relate or not.

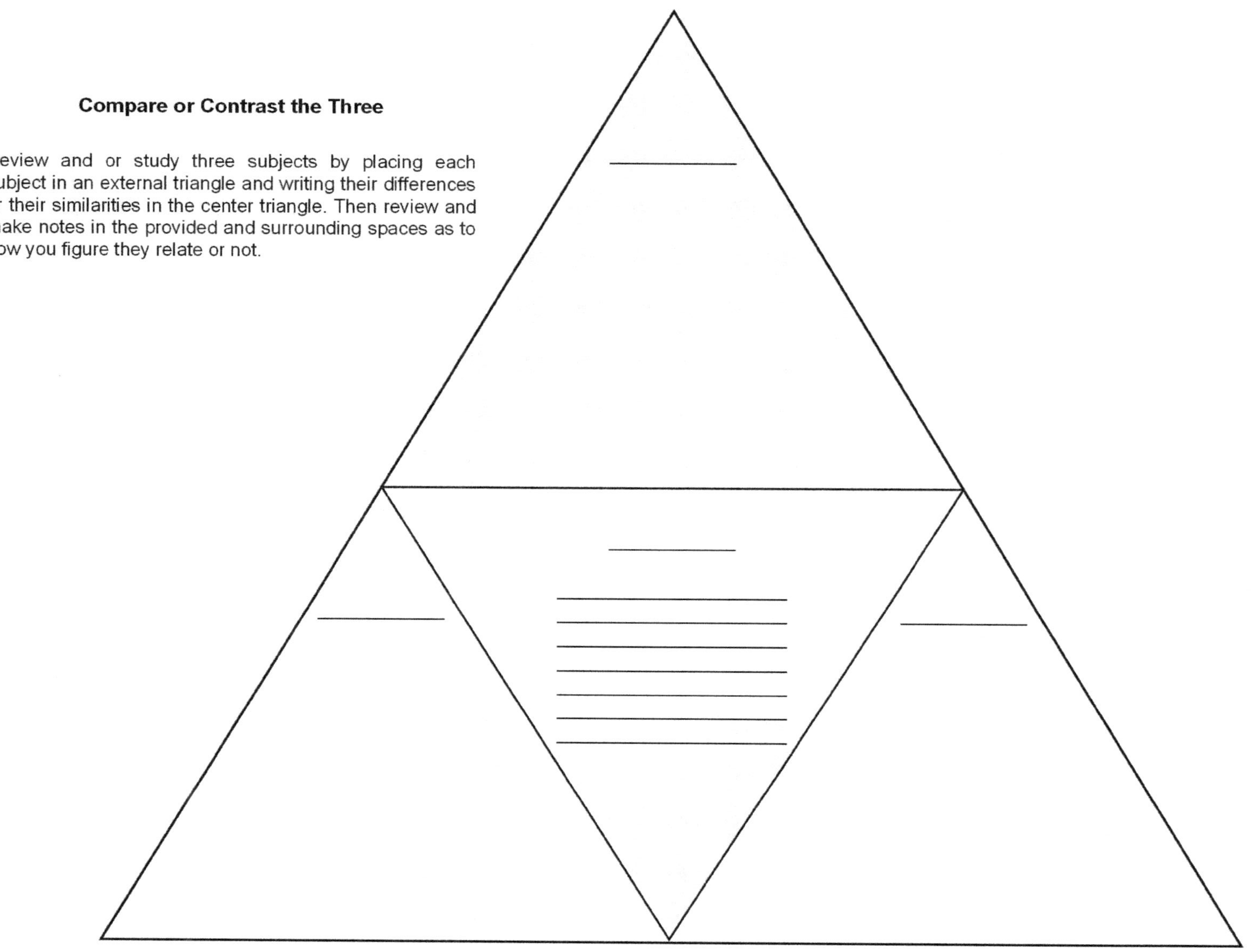

Questionnaire

1. How many meals a day do you eat?

2. Do you eat breakfast?

   a. If so, what does it consist of?

   b. What time do you eat?

3. Do you eat lunch?

   a. If so, what does it consist of?

   b. What time do you eat?

4. Do you eat dinner?

   a. If so, what does it consist of?

   b. What time do you eat?

5. Do you eat your meals alone or with others?

   a. If so, with whom?

6. Do you think you have good eating habits?

7. Do you exercise? If so, how often?

CPSIA information can be obtained
at www.ICGtesting.com
Printed in the USA
LVOW02s0106060516

486585LV00003B/9/P